THE CHRONIC OVERACHIEVER

A Personal Development Book for Women Navigating Challenges with Confidence

KASEY BOEHMER, PHD, MPH, NBC-HWC

▸ WISE INK ◂
MINNEAPOLIS, MN

ISBN-13: 978-1-63489-965-9
Library of Congress Catalog Number: 2025913654
Printed in the United States of America
First Printing: 2025
29 28 27 26 25 5 4 3 2 1

Cover and interior design by Emily Rodvold at lift-creative.com
Edited by Victoria Petelin and Susan McGrath
Proofread by Abbie Phelps and Karlee Steffanni
Production editing by Victoria Petelin
Images sourced from istockphoto.com

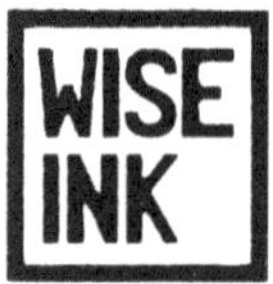

Wise Ink
PO Box 580195
Minneapolis, MN 55458-0195
wiseink.com

Wise Ink is a creative publishing agency for game-changers. Wise Ink authors uplift, inspire, and inform, and their titles support building a better and more equitable world. For more information, visit wiseink.com.

To order, visit itascabooks.com or kaseyboehmer.com. Reseller discounts available.

Contact Kasey Boehmer, PhD, MPH, NBC-HWC, at kaseyboehmer.com for speaking engagements, freelance writing projects, and interviews.

For Sweet Georgia Brown—our mum and memaw.
I hope there are books in heaven.

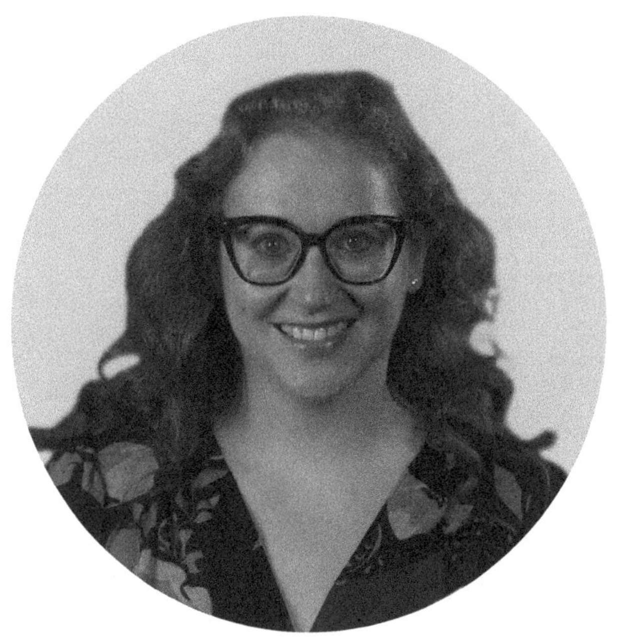

Kasey Boehmer, PhD, MPH, NBC-HWC, is an assistant professor of health services research and National Board-Certified Health and Wellness Coach. She is a faculty member in the Mayo Clinic Division of Nephrology and Hypertension and the Division of Health Care Delivery Research. She also serves as a lead researcher in the Knowledge and Evaluation Research (KER) Unit, leading the Minimally Disruptive Medicine Program. Her research and practice focus on supporting the capacity of patients, such that they can thrive despite living with chronic illnesses. She has authored or coauthored over sixty publications, including articles that outline the Theory of Patient Capacity, the ICAN Discussion Aid, and Capacity Coaching. Dr. Boehmer grounds her work in her experience of living with six chronic conditions herself and in her interactions with fellow patients.

DISCLAIMER

Many of the concepts in this book are based on peer-reviewed scientific literature and other trusted academic sources, which are cited in the text. However, this material is not meant to take the place of a consultation with a trained medical professional. The content of this book is for informational purposes only and is not intended to diagnose, treat, cure, or prevent any condition or disease. Please consider consulting a trusted healthcare practitioner to discuss specific struggles you may be experiencing.

The views expressed are the author's personal views and do not necessarily reflect the policy or position of Mayo Clinic.

THE ROLLER COASTER

The climb is terrifying
For the freefall that's coming
Fists clenched tight
How will you ever learn to enjoy the descent?

The certainty is terrifying
For the questioning that is coming
Legs trembling
How will you ever learn to walk upright?

The love is terrifying
For the heartbreak that is coming
Heart racing
How will you ever learn to proceed calmly?

The rainstorm is terrifying
For the drought that's yet to come
Skin shivering
How will you ever learn to dance in the rain?

The success is terrifying
For the failure that is inevitable
Mind racing
How will you ever learn to celebrate?

The symptoms are terrifying
For the uncertainty that they bring
Body revolting
How will you ever be normal again?

The lights others shine on you are terrifying
For the mirror they hold up shows all your imperfections
Contradictions revealed
How will you ever be just you?

But then the miracle of surrender happens
And the freefall becomes enjoyable
The questioning clarifies your ideas
The heartbreak means you truly loved

The drought brings resilience
The failure brings success
The symptoms bring meaning
The lights bring you into stardom

You see, everything you've ever been afraid of
Is exactly what you need
Right here, right now
The roller coaster awaits your embrace

TABLE OF CONTENTS

INTRODUCTION

I'm sitting in the driver's seat of my light-yellow 2006 Volkswagen Beetle, dressed in trendy business casual and smart flats, my red curls formed from air-dried scrunching. I'm in the parking garage at the Mall of America in Bloomington, Minnesota, looking out across the way at the giant building that takes you on an endless loop through tourism and retail paradise. I've just finished my eight-hour shift at Nordstrom, where I've been working for a few months since moving to Minnesota from Texas. There is a dam filled with tears hovering just above the lower lashes of my green eyes, held back since my earlier lunch break. Two and a half months earlier, I launched into the unknown, said goodbye to every single thing I'd ever known and loved, and left to pursue a dream of a college degree and the adult life a degree brought with it. Before leaving, I felt the deep tug of my intuition. Now—desperately lonely and crying in my car—all the certainty I had when I left Texas is gone. I begin to wonder, are my dreams too big? Will they crush me before I ever see their fruition? Am I ever going to find a place of belonging in this new place and stage in my life?

These questions are on my mind because when I arrived in Minnesota, it was nothing like I'd pictured in my mind. Most people I meet, at work or out and about, think it's weird that a seventeen-year-old girl left a perfectly good homelife for a place where she knows no one. Who does that for a dream? How could I be so certain I could pull it off? Despite my extroverted nature, no one is rushing to befriend me in my new home state. The rules of the game, this adulthood thing I've thrust myself into, are completely different and impenetrably opaque. Not a soul around is going to save me from that. I can either run back home to Texas or run forward into the unknown toward a college dream on the path I've laid out for myself. Only I can choose to quit or to endure the hard life lessons that feel like they are cracking at the very foundation of my confidence.

* * *

Flash forward approximately ten years to an early spring day in Minnesota in the year 2016. This time, I'm sitting on a green couch in the house I own with a dam of tears at the brim of my green eyes again. This time, I don't just feel miserable emotionally. My pelvis sears with a hot and tugging pain, only slightly dulled by the dose of pain medication taken a few hours prior. It's been months like this. Since the pain began, they've tried everything to figure out why it started. I've endured medical scans, bloodwork, physical exams, and even exploratory surgery without any definitive answers. In this moment, I am terrified that the decade of hard work I have put in to build the life of my dreams is going to be stripped away from me entirely because I am chronically ill. Back in 2006, I faced the hard work of pursuing my dreams past the depths of my loneliness, despair, and uncertainty. Here, a decade later, I've built a life that includes a family, one graduate degree in hand and another in progress, and a career path. That castle I've been building is actively crumbling before my eyes.

My medical team and I are beginning to coalesce around the idea that my symptoms might be from a chronic condition called interstitial cystitis, or bladder pain syndrome (IC/BPS). By now, I am well trained in medical terminology and research, which means that I know IC/BPS has a severe impact on many patients' quality of life, including their ability to maintain full-time employment.[1,2] I'm a wife and mother of a three-year-old, and my breadwinning abilities are important to my family. Equally important, my self-image as a career woman is a core identity. My biography is one of a hustling dream catcher who can overcome anything.

As I sit on my couch contemplating all of this mess, my sweet mother is in the kitchen doing my dishes because I cannot bear to get up now to do them. She has the energy that I don't. I lament, "I just want to be normal again." She answers with, "You will. Do you want me to pray with you?"

* * *

Mom was the strongest in faith of any person I'd ever met. She was not necessarily strictly religious, but rather she had a deep, connected spiritual faith that I am glad she passed on to me. She sat next to me on the couch and prayed with many more words than I can now recall, but what I do remember is her saying, "God, heal her in ways that only you can."

He didn't heal my bladder—I was indeed diagnosed with IC/BPS—but he healed my soul in a way that allowed me to take the hard parts of that journey and use them meaningfully in my work. I had been chronically ill my whole life—by age seven, I was diagnosed with severe and life-threatening allergies, asthma, and Wolff-Parkinson-White syndrome, a heart defect that causes very high heart rates to occur.

However, it was this new diagnosis of IC/BPS that suddenly made me realize that the work I was doing as a researcher dedicated to studying the ways to live well with chronic illness was intimately connected to my own story. And with that connection, I would be able to bring a unique voice and potential for change to the many problems that patients with chronic illness face every day. I can now, without difficulty, cross the terrain between the everyday work of managing chronic illnesses and the best scientific evidence to support those practices. I can also cross the terrain of a working mother in academia juggling a family, a career, and a chronically ill body, because after my IC/BPS diagnosis, I was also diagnosed with two autoimmune diseases, Sjögren's syndrome and mixed connective tissue disease.

None of these are visible when you see me, so I am someone who lives with what is sometimes described as "invisible disability." To physically function in my daily life, I take twelve prescription medications and five supplements every day. I must focus on getting enough sleep, exercise, and good nutrition, not just because they're good for me generally, but because if I don't, my symptoms increase in severity.

In addition to my lived experience, I have had considerable professional success. I am an assistant professor of health services research and a National Board–Certified Health and Wellness Coach (NBC-HWC) at a major academic medical center in the United States. I hold a master's in public health (MPH) and a PhD in nursing. I have authored over sixty publications on the topics of resilience, chronic illness self-management, patient capacity, and coaching in chronic illness. One of these publications puts forth a theory of patient capacity.[3] Simply put, this theory describes what it holistically takes for people living with chronic illness to thrive through the inevitable challenges chronic illness brings. As of 2025, this theory has been cited in 124 other academic publications. My work since 2016 has focused on how we help patients by increasing their capacity, not just to manage their conditions, but to live joyful lives. I coach patients to do just that as they navigate living with life-altering chronic illnesses.

Truthfully, it is a major challenge to balance my natural tendencies as a goal-getter with carefully managing my health. This is something that able-bodied people often take for granted. Yet, I have had success in my life and career despite that challenge. Now, I'm sharing with you the foundational lessons and practices I have learned to navigate the roller coaster of these challenges. It bears mentioning, however, that navigating these challenges is hard. Every time I've encountered hard things in life—some of my own choosing, like moving away from home at a young age, and some I never would have chosen, like chronic illness—I not only survived the experience, I grew from it. But growing is hard work.

Think about the challenge a seed encounters when it enters the soil and begins its growth trajectory. First it cracks, and then it breaks open completely. It starts growing downward, extending its roots below, before it grows upward and sprouts for the world to see. And once it begins its upward journey, it slowly unfurls. It bows its head before it rises. Not until that process is complete can it truly begin to spring toward the sun and the sky to reach its full potential. That's the way every transformative growth experience has felt walking through it. It felt like cracking open, sinking deeper into the depths of pain and frustration, and slowly rising back up to greet the sun above the soil. I can see now in hindsight that these periods of growth were required to get where I am today.

I know that hearing "it'll all work out" isn't particularly useful when you're in the middle of a tough time. That's why I have revisited those hard times I went through during my early adulthood to hopefully share some insights into both the emotions I had and the strategies I used during those times. These nuggets of resilience are what I lean into even now during new challenging seasons.

I call the strategies that I use "antidotes." According to Merriam-Webster, an antidote is "something that relieves, prevents, or counteracts." Sometimes, an antidote is a literal elixir that is consumed to counteract a poison, like a snakebite. Other times, an antidote is a carefully curated habit that keeps your eyes on your goals even when it feels like your world is crumbling around you. Obviously, I'm sharing the latter type of antidotes with you; please go to your nearest emergency room if you need a snakebite antidote.

You don't have to use these antidotes—all of them or any of them—but I hope you pause to consider them. Whether you live with chronic illness, are an overachiever just starting out, or are a busy parent trying to balance work, homelife, and some semblance of self-care, I think you will find something in the chapters ahead that will help.

This isn't going to be self-help in the usual sense of "if you just pulled yourself up by the bootstraps and got on with it, everything would be fine." Rather, we're going to model our approach after the seed forging its way ahead toward the light. Sometimes, the soil we're planted in is imperfect. There aren't enough nutrients within, or, worse, there are boulders in the way of our direct path upward. We're going to take real, imperfect life circumstances and talk about the ways in which we can navigate through them toward holistic health.

The book is divided into three sections that will help you navigate. In the first section, I will cover challenges of uncertainty and the fear of the unknown. These accompanied me during my earliest adulthood when I set off to forge my own path seventeen hours away from home by car, leaving behind everything I'd ever known. Overcoming your fear of the unknown means pushing outside your comfort zone.

The second section will focus on managing ambiguity and external challenges. While the early experiences of my adulthood were uncertain, the path from a high-school graduate to a college graduate was a well-defined one. As I exited my college years and moved into my career, things began to look a lot messier. That's because there is no right career development path, and usually there are some boulders in the way of the path you choose to take. Ultimately, you must persist through all the real-life distractions, negativity, and apathy that will consistently try to deter you from your path. Success is then stringing together a series of actions that move you forward, even if you don't feel prepared or motivated in the moment.

In the third and final section, we will discuss building a secure foundation for safety, joy, and progress as you move through life. Regardless of who we are, life is going to throw some very hard curveballs at us. These include family dynamics, acute or chronic illness, grief, and world-changing events like a pandemic. Even high achievers don't get a pass. The key to moving through these is to engage the foundational capacity that you build within yourself and within community. Here, I will draw upon my own personal experiences, as well as the experiences my team and I have summarized about the capacity to navigate life's toughest waters.

I am excited to share the stories that shaped me and the antidotes that I leaned on to navigate and find eventual success even in the hard times.

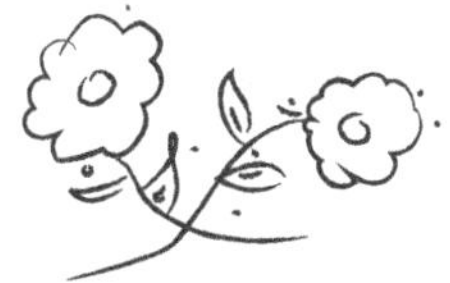

PART I

ANTIDOTES FOR

When You Question Your Decisions

When I was seventeen years old, living in a new state seventeen hours from home, following my dreams of a college degree, I had a breakdown in the parking lot of the mall I worked at. Before I left home, I was a wide-eyed dreamer who set out on a path I had chosen with no doubt it would work out. Faced with the new reality of loneliness without my family or friends and the real day-to-day work of making it on my own as an adult, I felt like I had made a terrible mistake. Suddenly, I was overwhelmed by the idea that maybe my dreams were too big to accomplish.

In this first month away from home, I could hear the fateful conversation between my parents and me in our living room. I had devised a plan to finish high school through distance learning (back then this was correspondence courses through postal mail), transfer from working at Nordstrom in my Dallas suburb to Nordstrom at the Mall of America, and then enroll at the University of Minnesota to pursue an undergraduate degree in political science. During the conversation where I shared these ideas, my dad immediately went into protective papa mode—in the best way possible—and voiced his concerns that sending me off into the world so far away at such a young age was absolutely bananas. My mom, in her calm yet firm way, shared her experience as a young woman, not allowed to leave home until she was married—at nineteen—to pursue a degree. She, having overcome that patriarchal notion, was now a mother with a master's degree and would not stand in my way of leaving. Instead, she would do whatever she could to support it.

With her blessing and willingness to convince my father, I had followed my completely uncharted path with a goal to enroll within a year or two at the University of Minnesota to pursue my undergraduate degree. While most people wondered if I'd considered the winter weather in Minnesota, I was drawn to the beautifully luscious summers and the autumn leaves that surrounded the downtown campus—and to the ice rinks, plentiful in Minnesota, as a former figure skater and hockey enthusiast.

Had I moved after finishing high school and started college right away, as an out-of-state resident, my undergraduate degree would have cost twice as much as it would if I were an in-state resident. While my family had resources for which I am grateful, the rate of tuition would have been a significant burden to our household. My education would need to be covered mostly by student loans, and I knew just enough about finances to know that reducing the amount of money taken in loans made good financial sense. And herein lies the reason I decided to pack my bags, finish my senior year of high school at a distance, and work at Nordstrom in Minnesota until I had saved some money and could enroll as an in-state resident.

So, in the summer of 2006 I said my goodbyes to my family and friends, and I left early one August morning with all my things in a U-Haul truck bound for Minnesota. My dad drove the truck and stayed for a few weeks until my seventeenth birthday to help me settle in. Surprisingly, it wasn't particularly difficult from a logistics perspective to live on my own as a seventeen-year-old. My parents cosigned my lease and my bank accounts. No one really asked any questions otherwise, except when I needed to seek medical care. In such cases, the treating healthcare team would call my parents for consent to care for me.

Regardless of how certain I was in my decisions up until that moment, when my dad closed the door to leave me in my apartment alone for the very first time, I panicked. I thought maybe if I opened my door and ran to the parking lot before he could leave, I could just say this had been a nice try, but I wanted to go home.

I didn't do that. So instead, I met loneliness for the first time. Just like the newly planted seed, I was now deep in the soil, but not ready to grow upward. Instead, I would experience painfully breaking open and setting roots. That first night was just the beginning of the emotional whirlwind I went through. I was homesick, grieving the loss of a life that was comfortable, in shock, and mystified all at the same time. Five days a week, I would go to work, and I remember on every single break I would go to Caribou Coffee and call my mom, desperate to hear her voice. She never pushed me to stay; she knew I was stubborn enough to see out my own dreams. I was cut from the same cloth as she. Instead, she just listened to me and provided me with what wisdom she could when she could.

Sometimes I was desperate for the positivity boost she would give me, and sometimes I was desperate to hear the monotony of her day. These calls felt to me like curling up with my favorite cozy blanket when it's cold, raining, and dreadful out. And then I would get through the second half of my workday, and when my shift ended I would sit in the parking lot and cry. This went on for a couple of months before my seedling began to transition to the journey upward toward new life.

Slowly, I could see the glimmer of light and hope, just like the seed breaking through the topsoil. Each new day, these glimmers were brief snapshots of the person I was becoming. This person was someone who was still the dreamer but was now also taking action toward her independence and future self. Truthfully, I think the reason I didn't give up on myself when my dad left, or every day after when I wanted to go home, was that I knew I would be letting myself down.

I'd long fought against the odds—as a chronically ill kid, to get to a point where I was healthy enough to be an athlete. And once I was an athlete—a figure skater—I'd spend three hours a day throwing myself up into the air only to fall hard to the ice repeatedly for the chance to just once figure out the physics of landing on a millimeters-thick blade. I didn't just give up after throwing myself up in the air once or at a single practice. I did it repeatedly until I figured it out. I'd never let myself down before, and I wasn't about to start now.

Even though the question, "Have I made a terrible mistake?" echoed in my head often those first few months, the question of

"Who are you if you give up?" provided a powerful counterargument. I didn't want to be a quitter. I never went back. I never quit the journey. Ultimately, I see now that my ability to stick it out was dependent on two key factors. Those were 1) proactively and intentionally shaping my identity of who I wanted to become, and 2) nurturing meaningful connections.

Let's look at how those two ideas worked in action.

PROACTIVELY AND INTENTIONALLY SHAPE YOUR IDENTITY.

That first hard year, every time I got into my car after a work shift, I turned on a song called "She Said," by Brie Larson. The chorus went:

> I know it's a long way down
> But you can't walk the wire
> For anybody else
> I might hit the ground
> But at least I'll have a story to tell
> She said, I gotta find out for myself

Intertwined in this song was an identity: an independent, trailblazing female who even if she fell was going to try walking the tightrope herself. This identity felt very in alignment with the person I was when I chose to move to Minnesota, but once I had arrived felt very far away. In my new home state, I felt lost, alone, and uncertain. It took daily reminders that I was the independent woman and not the fearful girl.

This song was that daily reminder for me, and it generated in me a feeling that I desperately needed to hold on to: conviction. When you step up to face the uncertainty, you too will need to purposefully cultivate an identity that you are moving toward. To create this identity, you will need to find ways in which you can remind yourself of what that new person looks like and thinks like. You also will need to generate what it feels like to be that person even if it is counter to how you feel in the other moments of your day. The reason cultivating those feelings is important is that they drive our actions. If you feel meek, you take actions that shrink you.

If you feel convicted to become someone bigger and bolder, you act in ways that will grow you, just like water and nutrients feed the seedling as it journeys upward.

Music has unique properties as a method to cultivate your new identity. Specifically, it can help create a calmer, more centered version of yourself. This is because music activates aspects of your brain that are responsible for releasing hormones that make you feel pleasure and motivation as well as calm your stress responses.[1] When music interventions are used with patients living with chronic illness, researchers have found that they reduce depression and anxiety, and improve mood and quality of life.[2] For these reasons, I highly recommend incorporating purposeful music listening as part of your daily practices. However, you may also choose other reminders of who you want to be in this new phase of life. For example, you could place a piece of art somewhere you will see it every day, wear a special piece of jewelry daily, or even get a tattoo.

The key is to have one or more daily reminders that spark a continued feeling, like conviction, that will provide motivation to keep you moving toward the actions you need to take to be successful.

KNOW AND CULTIVATE YOUR MOST MEANINGFUL CONNECTIONS.

As you move into new territory, whether that be metaphorically or physically, your social support is critical. However, if you have made a big transition, you likely haven't yet established the connections in your new place to give you the emotional or practical support you need. It's important to know who your support team is and how you can reach them in your new and uncertain situation.

For me, when I was desperately uncertain of the big life choices I had made, I called my mother. In my opinion, no one was as wise about life and about what was good for me as my mother. She was my closest friend and confidant for twenty-eight years. No one believed in me and my abilities and strengths like my mama did. When I first left home, she would periodically send me little care packages—like a bar of chocolate, a card with a note and $20 inside, or a little stuffed animal that said goofy things to make me laugh. Mom was my ultimate cheerleader and a source of practical and financial support when I felt stuck.

For you, it may not be a parent that is your go-to person. Instead, it may be a different family member or a friend you've left behind. The most important thing is that, when you feel isolated and alone because of a big decision you made, this lifeline helps you remember that you are not actually alone in this.

I also want to impart to you that no matter how helpful your lifeline is, you need to cultivate new relationships as well. This is particularly important if you've moved to a new place—city, state, or country. Within a year's time, you want to have at least a handful of people with whom you are building friendships.

A helpful way to think about this might be to consider who you enjoy conversing or sharing hobbies with, are in similar life stages as, or could call in case of an emergency. When I had just moved, I sought out other people who were working in the same mall to meet for coffee or lunch on a break to talk and learn more about their lives. During my off time, I would go to the rink to skate or watch a hockey game and strike up a conversation with others there who had the love of ice in common with me. I also spent a lot of time at the nearby coffee shop studying. Coffee shops have the same group of people—the "regulars"—show up day in and day out to work on their goals and dreams. If you're a goal-getter, those might be your new BFFs. Indeed, places can facilitate social growth and belonging. Researchers have found that community places where patrons visit for shared purposes and social engagement create a stronger sense of community and are more important in their lives than noncommunity places. For example, a gym where visitors go to a group exercise class every week with the same group of people is more likely to play an important role in an individual's life than a large shopping center where visits are irregular and driven by consumption of goods, not socialization.[3]

Finally, remember that we often cannot be everything to someone, and therefore, we should not expect a single person to be everything for us. We need a web of people who have different roles in our life, but each relationship we pursue should be meaningful in some way. We shouldn't underestimate the significance of varying levels of friendship or care. When we feel lonely, we often imagine meeting someone with whom we can find deep connection. Practically, a variety of levels of connection, from close confidant to those who can provide you a car ride in a pinch, are valuable.

In scientific literature, the collections of familial ties, friendships, and acquaintanceships we have are referred to as social ties. They exist on a gradient of closeness that can be described as weak, moderate, or strong. Different individuals may have different breakdowns of these relationships in their lives. For example, in a study of people living with chronic illnesses, about half of their relationships were strong ties. The remainder of their social network was characterized as moderate ties (34 percent) and weak ties (16 percent). However, all social ties had some role to play in their everyday lives and illness management.[4] This underscores that when we move to a new place, establishing a broad network of relationships, regardless of whether they become your new bestie, is critically important.

The community you foster, both in-person and at a distance, is important to finding certainty in your decisions as you develop your individual identity. Good relationships help reinforce the best parts of our identity as we move forward. Find your people, find yourself.

REFLECTION PROMPTS:

- Who do you need to reach out to right now for support during your current situation?
- What emotion do you need to conjure to overcome the uncertainty that you face right now?
- What actions would you take if you consistently felt this way?
- What song can generate that emotion you need right now to overcome this challenge?

"Find your people, find yourself."

ANTIDOTES FOR

When You're Scared

I live with six chronic illnesses. The first one I knew about was severe and life-threatening allergies. As a result, one of the ever-present things I fear is accidentally ingesting a peanut product and ultimately dying from that mistake. This has been a pervasive fear in my life since I became aware of my allergy, probably around age three or four, when I almost died in the car on the way to the hospital following airborne exposure to peanut butter. I remember sitting in the front seat of Mom's red Pontiac Grand Am. I remember her looking from me to the road and back again repeatedly. I could see the panic in her eyes, and I could feel she was speeding. I could tell she was running red lights. I remember that seemingly less and less air was available to my lungs. I don't remember arriving at the hospital, and I don't remember what happened once we got there. All I know is that I survived.

After this incident, I stayed safe in childhood mostly due to controlled environments and diligence on both my part and my parents' part; friends always came over to my house, not me to theirs. God bless my mother for putting up with a lot of screaming girls simply to keep me safe. Once I went out into the real world, though, not all things could be so controlled. Unfortunately, despite all the precautions I take to ask about peanuts at restaurants, read food labels, and secure peanut-safe travel arrangements, I've still been exposed multiple times in adulthood.

My greatest risk for exposure comes during travel. I had never set foot on an airplane until I was sixteen years old, simply because the level of exposure risk on airplanes was too great. In today's times, certain airlines don't serve peanuts, and I am able to travel periodically for work. Yet, the level of precautions I must take are far outside the norm of what folks without allergies think about. I ensure that I am on a peanut-free airline, have at least three Epi-Pens and twelve Benadryl tablets with me, bring written materials about my allergy in the native language of anywhere I am traveling outside the United States, and carry backup snacks to share with any passengers next to me that happened to bring a peanut-containing snack so that I can kindly ask them to put their peanut-containing food away.

Even so, leaving home leaves me with a sense of dread, especially if I overthink what will happen if I inadvertently consume a peanut product. Imagine this fear spiral . . .

> *What happens if I am on board the plane and I have a reaction? Will the medication on board stabilize me enough to get me back on the ground? How long will I be dealing with a reaction midair? My lord, at least three hours of this journey is over the ocean with no landing spot in sight. Once I get off the flight, how far to a hospital? How will I explain insurance coverage if I am unconscious? How will I communicate what is in my very complex medical record if I am at a hospital that doesn't have the same electronic health record storage as the hospital I go to? How will anyone know to call my family to tell them what is happening if I am unconscious? How long will they go without hearing from me, making them panic that something has happened to me in flight? What happens to my family if I die from this exposure?*

If that went through your head on a regular basis, would you want to leave the comfort of home ever?

Here's the problem with that anxiety spiral keeping me home: the only way that I'll ever get past fear is to take action while I'm still afraid. You grow because you choose to do the things that scare you repeatedly until you develop your own alternative storyline of how you make it work.

Here's how I have done that.

ANSWER YOUR BRAIN'S MOST ANXIETY-PROVOKING QUESTIONS.

In this instance, think about your worst-case scenario and write it down. Then answer your brain's natural "then what?!?" response to at least five questions.

To walk you through this, I will continue to use my worst-case scenario of ingesting a peanut product while away from home. Remember, the underlying fear is that I die and don't make it home to my family. However, the thoughts that are driving me to think that I might die and not make it home are actually my brain's questions about the worst-case scenarios that it doesn't have the answer to. Because my brain doesn't have the answer to them, it assumes that if I ingest the peanut, it's game over. So here we go, five questions of my brain spiral:

1. **What happens if you are midair on an international flight?**
   Answer: I need to tell airline personnel I am having a reaction and administer medication.
2. **How much medication would you need to support yourself through a reaction to get you safely to a hospital?**
   Answer: I need to discuss this with my doctor and ensure I have adequate supplies on board with me. I also need security personnel to know I have my doctor's oversight, which might require a medical letter.
3. **What if you're traveling on an airline where the staff won't understand you verbally telling them you are having a reaction?**
   Answer: I need a written form of communication in the language they will understand.
4. **What if you're landing in a country that isn't the United States and you need healthcare when you get to the ground?**
   Answer: I need to find a hospital that will accept my insur-

ance coverage, which I can probably research in advance before any emergency occurs.

5. **What happens if I have a reaction and need to communicate to my family that an emergency has occurred while traveling?**
Answer: I need to discuss with my family in advance what their communication preferences would be in such a hypothetical situation.

My fears about peanut exposure are well founded. My worst-case scenario has actually happened. With about two hours left over the ocean on a trip, I was accidentally given food with peanut oil in it. However, it wasn't game over because I had a game plan. I knew how much medicine I could take, and I had it next to me on board. I had written communication about what was occurring to share with the flight attendant. I was able to get safely onto the ground and avoid hospitalization afterward. Had I not done the exercise of rehearsing the worst-case scenario in my head, I might never have even faced the fear enough to get in an airplane, or, once I was in the situation, I would have truly panicked.

When we experience fear or anxiety, our bodies produce sensations that cue us to move away from the thing we are afraid of, regardless of whether the threat is a real danger or not. When you are afraid, you might notice sensations like sweaty palms, a racing heart, or the inability to focus on anything else.[1] These are your body's cues to run away from whatever danger it's going to encounter. While this was evolutionarily useful for running away from bears in the wild, it's less helpful in a world where many things seem scary, yet we want or need to confront them.

So what about your worst-case scenario? Maybe it isn't life and death, but it feels very scary, like making a presentation for the first time in front of a classroom on a topic you don't feel very comfortable with. The task is straightforward, but you're terrified that you could forget everything, completely embarrass yourself, bomb the presentation, and begin the descent into failing your entire college career, leaving you to move back home to your parents' basement. If your brain doesn't have answers to the spiral questions, it assumes game over, and to your parents' basement you go. In this instance, five spiraling questions might sound like:

1. **What if I must present first?**
   Answer: I need to mentally prepare that this could happen and think of ways that I might use that to my advantage. Can I connect with the audience quickly by making them laugh?
2. **What if I forget what I'm supposed to say in the middle of the presentation?**
   Answer: I must either have notes that will help me pick up my train of thought or have rehearsed enough times that I can improv it.
3. **What if I get horribly sweaty hands because I'm so nervous?**
   Answer: I need to wear something that can conceal my sweaty palms, like dark colors.
4. **What if I get dry mouth and I can't keep talking?**
   Answer: I can bring water up with me to the podium, pause quickly to take a sip, then continue. I should rehearse this too.
5. **What if the professor asks me a question that I don't know the answer to?**
   Answer: I can have a classmate help me by asking me questions after I do a rehearsal presentation with them to practice answering on the fly. I need to also have a gracious way to state I don't know the answer but do know how I can go about finding it.

By answering these questions in advance, you help your brain know that even if the worst-case scenario occurs, you have a plan. You have the skills to figure it out in the moment. Not every worst-case scenario can be known in advance, but the ones that are ultimately causing you anxiety in this very present moment are ones that can cause your brain to conjure up and imagine things going down in a horrific death spiral sort of way.

GIVE IT TO GOD.

Fear and avoidance can also diminish our quality of life and willingness to try new things. An example of this is our fear of physical pain. As someone who lives with chronic pain conditions, I can certainly say a pain flare-up is not one bit fun. Mine can leave me so achy, every movement feels like my joints need an oil can or that my pelvis has an anvil on top of it. However, focusing on my inability to control the pain rather than trying a variety of strategies to manage it, or avoiding activities because there is a chance they will worsen the pain (without having tried them to determine if this is true), diminishes my enjoyment of life and further limits my daily activities. In over three hundred studies looking at how we process pain, research has shown that there are significant correlations between feeling fearful or not in control of our pain experience and feeling emotions such as depression and anxiety, or how impactful we feel our disability is on our everyday lives.[2]

So, while the logical approach of answering at least five "what-if" questions certainly decreases my fears, it isn't always enough to pull me completely out of my anxiety brought on by whatever situation I am dealing with at the moment. Inevitably, my brain will find a way to scream, "I FOUND A NEW SCENARIO FOR HOW EVERYTHING CAN FALL APART!" More often than I'd like to admit, this will wake me from sleep in a dead panic.

In those moments, even when I have done my very best to allay my brain's fears, I can't offer it much more than "yeah, that might happen." And when that is the best I have to offer, I have a saying I use like a mantra: "Give it to God."

Regardless of your spiritual perspective, I find it extremely hard to navigate the difficult day-to-day living without thinking that there isn't some higher power that is helping me out. Belief in a higher power, for me, goes a long way in helping me come to acceptance. I believe there are things that I cannot explain in the moment but somehow work out for the best in the long run.

When I give something over to God, I am very explicit about this. I pray. I say something like, "God, I am terribly scared that [insert spiraling thought here] will happen. Please help me remember that you take this fear on for me and are working things out in the best possible plan."

Another tactic for giving my fears to God, particularly when I am in my waking hours, is to use my anxious energy to do something good or productive. So, if I can't sit still because that means I will be alone and silent with my thoughts, I can do the dishes for my family or I can go play outside with my kids. If I am scared about my finances, maybe I invest my time in researching ways to improve that situation or in volunteering for a charitable organization. Even in the absence of funds, I can gift precious time. There is always a pathway to use the nervous energy I have for good rather than directing it in an unkind way at others or making myself feel physically awful with dread.

What would it look like if you sat with your anxiety and captured its energy to be used for good? Instead of channeling that pent-up negative energy into a quarrel or self-spiral, you could clean your house, prepare a speech, or serve your community. Through such behavior we use our fear to create action that is going to make the world a better place. The anxiety and negative emotions may not go away, but at least they will be channeled into good.

REFLECTION PROMPTS:

- When it comes to your goals and dreams, where is fear stopping you in its tracks? What is your brain's "game-over" scenario?
- What are your five "what-if" questions and their respective answers?
- When you think about your fears, what do you want your alternative storyline to be? What small action can you take in the next week that is in opposition to your fear?
- Who gets the worst of you when you're anxious? How might you productively use that fearful energy instead?

"You grow because you choose to do the things that scare you repeatedly until you develop your own alternative storyline of how you make it work."

ANTIDOTES FOR

Distractions

In my opinion, distraction is the number one challenge you will face in getting from where you are now to where you want to be. This is something I was barely beginning to contend with in my early adulthood. However, now you can quite literally distract your life away with the steady stream of readily available entertainment, notifications, and news you can find in our everyday environment. In many ways, I feel sorry for my generation and all those that follow, because it wasn't always this way.

I am a millennial, and we are the first generation to know social media. When I left home at sixteen to set off for Minnesota, the digital landscape looked very different from what it is now. I didn't have a smartphone, and social media was still rudimentary. I came of age using Myspace. The real digital revolution, or maybe we should call it distraction doomsday, was in 2008, when Facebook launched its iPhone-based app. Suddenly you could be hanging out with your friends in real life while also having digital friends in your pocket. I left home at a time when I had to sit with my uncomfortable aloneness and had plenty of time to focus on my goals in my new home. I didn't have to constantly contend with distraction nagging at me. I worked, I studied, and I watched some basic cable television. I sat alone in restaurants without scrolling on a smartphone because all I could do was send SMS text messages on my old-school cell phone.

I am not a tech scrooge. I use my smartphone and tablet often now, as do the rest of my family. And although I try to limit my social media consumption, there are aspects of social media that are arguably good. Today we can connect with people all over the world—some we have met in real life and some we have not—through social media. People who feel isolated in their physical community can find digital community. Maybe this could have been helpful in making me feel not so alone at the time I left home. But, y'all, these societal goods have come at a monumental cost; we are missing out on the lives right in front of us. While I certainly do not think that we can or would want to rid our world of these life-changing technological advances, I need you to hear: *if you do not cultivate a self-awareness around your digital consumption, you are at risk of never accomplishing your goals.*

Our digital landscape is dangerous because these innovations are so embedded in our current culture that choosing something else requires us to exert active energy to do so. Digital distraction is harmful because if you feel uncomfortable—maybe you're sad, angry, or lonely—you can avoid ever having to address that negative emotion because you get to distract it away. And here's the thing: your goals, whether it's that degree, that promotion, that family, that car, that house, you name it, are going to require long, hard, consistent effort, and an onslaught of uncomfortable emotions. It is much more enjoyable to scroll social media or binge-watch the next Netflix series. Pretty soon, those hours you set aside to make meaningful progress toward your dreams are gone. And they're gone to absolutely nothing.

I would argue that while some digital distraction can be a reasonable downtime activity, when these distractions begin to pull us away from accomplishing our goals, they become something more serious. Researchers define problematic internet use as the "use of the internet that creates psychological, social, school and/or work difficulties in a person's life."[1] Certain internet activities are more strongly associated with this phenomenon, including general surfing (aka, following that rabbit hole after you look up one thing), shopping, and social networking.[2] Further, problematic internet use has been associated with declines in cognitive performance, including decision-making and working memory.[3] Those two brain functions are incredibly important in making daily progress in life.

Contributing to our digital distraction and problematic internet use is that online environments are sometimes intentionally structured to be addictive, as this maximizes the time a person stays engaged on a platform.[3] Build that tech development strategy upon our natural tendency to want to distract ourselves from hard things, and you've got a major challenge to overcome in progressing toward your goals.

What actions can you take to minimize digital distraction? Here are some of the things I have found helpful.

TIME TRACKING TO CULTIVATE SELF-AWARENESS.

To start, there are digital methods by which you can track your time. For example, all smartphones track your screen time automatically. However, looking at lumped data like hours of screen time per day alone isn't always granular enough to nail down your distraction landscape. For example, screen time might tell you how much you spent on social media apps, but if you use social media for work and home, the minutes spent are combined. Additionally, it doesn't tell you anything about how you feel in the moment that you drift into distracted mode instead of focused mode. And if you look back a few days later, you might not recall what exactly lulled you into two straight hours of scrolling. Did you drift there because you worked too many minutes straight and your brain was desperate for a break? Or was it because you had an uncomfortable conversation with your best friend and you were desperate to escape into distraction? This is why I recommend a brief analog strategy to truly understand how you spend your time.

While I have heard other personal development speakers talk about variations on this activity, I personally credit learning this time-tracking activity to Chalene Johnson, as an activity of her 30-Day Push Challenge, many years ago. I enacted this advice, and it totally changed my understanding of how to organize my days. Those I have mentored have similarly found it impactful in their quest toward an intentional life.

To assist you, I've prepared a template for you to use the next two weeks to track your time and activities. You can download it from **www.kaseyboehmer.com**. You can see a one-day example of the time tracking template on page 33 of this book. Here's how to use it. At the top of each hour on your template, write down what you did in the past hour. Note also how you felt during that hour, such as tired, hurried, focused, energized, engaged, present, or overwhelmed. Be short but specific and include anything that interrupted you, such as a quick ten-minute scroll through Instagram or an unexpected five-minute phone call. You may also want to jot down other things in the notes section at the end of each week, like where you were working each day—such as your home, your office, or a coffee shop—and any other information that seems pertinent, like how you slept the night before. You may also want to add into the notes any particularly salient events on the days that may be out of the norm. Include anything you find relevant to your time management each day—ultimately, this exercise is for you to get to know you.

For example, you might write in the Monday, 8 a.m., section, "Activities: answered 34 emails. Feeling: engaged." Or 3 p.m., "Activities: writing science paper, 10 min. social scroll. Feeling: sluggish." Each time you reflect on your previous hour, it should take you no more than one to two minutes to jot down these reflections.

After you have your two weeks of data, take time to sit and review them. Here are some things to think about. Notice any patterns about what times and places you're most likely to describe yourself as energized, productive, or engaged. Likewise, pay attention to times of the day when you're most likely to distract yourself from the present moment. See if you can spot what kind of day leads into a night where you are engaged and enjoy time with your friends or family. What did you do during the day on a night you slept well compared to a night that you tossed and turned? When do you feel confident and motivated versus self-loathing and critical? Pay attention to how your activities impact your behaviors—positively or negatively.

Once you have this data and your reflections, the next step is to use this data to purposefully reorganize your day and your activities to create and support the most intentional you. Intention is the opposite of distraction. Don't expect the first reorganization attempt to be perfect. This is going to require some experimentation, and we expect many experiments will fail. We learn from them and use them to try the next iteration. There are a few key things to include in your structured day to ensure you are living life intentionally rather than distracted.

First, map out your *power hours*. In your patterns, you likely have picked up that there are a couple hours of your day where you are naturally prone to productivity. Those two power hours you should seek to preserve, at least a few days a week, at all costs. For me, my typical power hours are 9 to 11 a.m. I try to ensure that at least a few days a week, there are no meetings occurring during that time and I leave my email turned off. I put my phone on do-not-disturb, and I power through activities that take significant brain power, writing, or creating. Now, power hours for me are part of my workday. In college, they were for studying. One of those may be true for you, or maybe your power hours are when you work on your side hustle. Whatever your dreams are, your power hours are intended to get you one step closer to them.

Second, pinpoint your *connection hours*. These are the hours in which you connect with the people most important to you in your life. For me, this is the time I spend with my family—primarily my husband, two kids, and dad. Usually, it is on evenings and weekends. However, if your power hours are during evenings, then you may need different connection hours.

Finally, determine your *sleep hours*. You cannot run on empty all the time. Matthew Walker, PhD and expert sleep scientist, discusses in his book *Why We Sleep* that after nineteen hours awake, your reaction abilities are no better than someone who is legally drunk.[4] Additionally, chronic sleep deprivation in small doses is equivalent to big chunks of unrested time. For example, four hours of sleep six days in a row is equivalent in terms of functioning to going without sleeping for twenty-four hours. To put this in perspective, that means the sleep you skimped on for the exam you crammed for or the project you just put in extra hours for all week long has left you as unsafe in reaction abilities as a drunk person. You may, like many people, try to tell me or convince yourself that you really don't need that much sleep. You're fine with five hours.

Most likely, you're not. The number of people who need less than seven to nine hours per night is about one in one hundred, but I guarantee there is a much larger percentage of people who think they fall into this category.

Therefore, through this time tracking and subsequent schedule alteration, try to truly identify your ideal amount of sleep if you don't know it already. For me, I function best with eight or nine hours, but I absolutely must average at least seven hours a night. However many hours you require, you need at least one additional hour in bed to get that amount. If you need eight hours of sleep, you need to be in your bed for nine hours. This is because we naturally wake up throughout the night, even when we don't realize it. There are various tech solutions available to see exactly how many minutes are consumed by restless time in bed, but the analog solution of adding one hour to your ideal sleep amount should do the trick.

To summarize, once you finish this activity, you should understand how to build your days with intention, and you should have three pillars in your days: power hours, connection hours, and sleep hours. No matter what level of overachiever you are, you only get twenty-four hours per day to slot these three core activities into. The habit of looking back on what you were able to do with those twenty-four hours helps you realistically start to predict how much you can fit into any given week. It's important that you plan the approximate amount of work that you can actually accomplish—barring any major catastrophes like an urgent health issue. This is important because our brain gives us a lot of negative feedback on the tasks we didn't accomplish—far more than it gives us positive feedback for the ones we did. By preparing for your week with realistic expectations, you will end up checking off more on your to-do list than not. This prevents your brain from telling you things like "you should have completed that sixth task," or "you're so inefficient, so-and-so would have done all of her to-do list." Rather, you'll feel accomplished, content, and more motivated to plan the next week ahead.

DISCIPLINE YOUR DISTRACTIONS.

It's one thing to plan your days; it's another thing to actually stick to the plan. Discipline gets a bad rap because it is associated with what our parents did when they put their foot down. Yet, for most of us, our parents or other adults who played a role in raising us didn't put their foot down because they enjoyed it. Honestly, as a parent, putting your foot down is a lot harder than just letting your tiny human run wild. Parents use discipline because they want good things for their offspring and the other kids in their community. Discipline is part of kids' development, not a detriment to it.

Same goes for you and me—discipline is part of our development, not a detriment to it. Whatever your goals are, they cannot be reached without discipline. That means turning off the TV, silencing the social media, sometimes saying no to that unneeded nap, skipping the night out. Please understand that I am not saying you never get to do these things. We shouldn't be working nonstop, and balance is important. However, I am saying that when you say you will do something in pursuit of your goals, you do them. You do not give in to distractions. *What you want will only show up if YOU keep showing up.* And showing up takes discipline.

Here are a few key distraction-fighting disciplines you can use.

1. **Screen time limits:** If you know that certain apps on your phone tend to pull you into distraction mode, use your settings to put a limit on how long you can be on those daily. For example, you can set a time limit that will kick you out of your social media apps if you have been on them more than thirty minutes for the day. (If you're regularly using social and haven't tried this before, it will be scary to see how fast thirty minutes goes by.)
2. **Notifications off:** You can turn off any app's ability to send you notifications. I recommend that only critical apps be allowed to send notifications (e.g., text messaging, phone calls).
3. **Do not disturb:** During your power, connection, and sleep

hours, if your phone is with you, use "do not disturb." You can set this mode on your phone to ensure that people can reach you in case of emergencies. For example, I can set it so that if day care or my husband calls me, it always rings through.

4. **Checklists:** I personally am much better at staying on task if I have a list of key things to do and can feel the satisfaction of marking them off. I don't put together a list that is a mile long, but rather two to three priorities that I want to make sure I get done for the day.
5. **Share your goals:** Tell a few key people what you're working on and working toward. Accountability makes it easier to say yes to the activities you need to be disciplined in seeing through. Saying yes to your goals sometimes means saying no to Sunday Funday, but when you have someone who is expecting you to make progress, it makes being disciplined a bit easier.

REFLECTION PROMPTS:

- What distractions do you lean into when things get hard? Is it social media, shopping, eating, or something else?
- Of power, connection, and sleep hours, which do you need to pay attention to most as you work on your intentionality?
- Which distraction-fighting discipline do you want to try? When will you put it into action?

RESOURCES:

Two-week time tracking worksheet available at **www.kaseyboehmer.com.**

SUNDAY

TIME	ACTIVITIES	FEELING
6 a.m.		
7 a.m.		
8 a.m.		
9 a.m.		
10 a.m.		
11 a.m.		
12 p.m.		
1 p.m.		
2 p.m.		
3 p.m.		
4 p.m.		
5 p.m.		
6 p.m.		

NOTES

FRIDAY

TIME	ACTIVITIES	FEELING
6 a.m.		
7 a.m.		
8 a.m.		
9 a.m.		
10 a.m.		
11 a.m.		

SATURDAY

TIME	ACTIVITIES	FEELING
6 a.m.		
7 a.m.		
8 a.m.		
9 a.m.		
10 a.m.		

WEDNESDAY

TIME	ACTIVITIES	FEELING
6 a.m.		
7 a.m.		
8 a.m.		
9 a.m.		
10 a.m.		
11 a.m.		
12 p.m.		
1 p.m.		
2 p.m.		
3 p.m.		
4 p.m.		
5 p.m.		
6 p.m.		
7 p.m.		
8 p.m.		
9 p.m.		

THURSDAY

TIME	ACTIVITIES	FEELING
6 a.m.		
7 a.m.		
8 a.m.		
9 a.m.		

MONDAY

TIME	ACTIVITIES	FEELING
6 a.m.		
7 a.m.		
8 a.m.		
9 a.m.		
10 a.m.		
11 a.m.		
12 p.m.		
1 p.m.		
2 p.m.		
3 p.m.		
4 p.m.		
5 p.m.		
6 p.m.		
7 p.m.		
8 p.m.		
9 p.m.		

TUESDAY

TIME	ACTIVITIES	FEELING
6 a.m.		
7 a.m.		
8 a.m.		
9 a.m.		
10 a.m.		
11 a.m.		
12 p.m.		
1 p.m.		
2 p.m.		
3 p.m.		
4 p.m.		
5 p.m.		
6 p.m.		
7 p.m.		
8 p.m.		
9 p.m.		

"Intention is the opposite of distraction."

ANTIDOTES FOR

Losing Yourself

Like any young individual setting out, I found myself in a relationship early in my college years. What I wish I had known then is that to have a successful partnership, you both must first know how to independently be yourselves well. If you are not clear on who you are independent of another person, you can easily fall into the trap of co-depending on the other person as a stand-in for your own likes, hopes, dreams, and desires.

I think you're particularly in danger of this occurring in your first relationship outside of your home of origin. The reason for this concern is that, for many people, until the time of moving out, you're somewhat integrated into family life—whether that is a positive or a negative experience. When you leave that family of origin and set out independently, it can feel very bewildering to be on your own. Suddenly, you can choose whatever you want to eat for dinner that night. You don't have to consider anyone else when picking out a movie. In that slightly uncomfortable space, as humans, we may naturally want to fill it rather than settling into our own rhythm of life.

I consider myself lucky—I had to survive the emotional hurricane of a serious relationship that ultimately dissolved only once. Following that relationship, I began dating my now-husband of thirteen years. What I can see on the other side of that breakup and my now-successful marriage is that in my previous relationship, I lost myself, while in my marriage I am wholly my own person, with a husband who is wholly his own person too. I now know that what makes you whole will never be found outside of yourself.

I can see past events that indicated these truths. For example, New Year's Eve in my second year living in Minnesota, I was home visiting family in Texas. I was at a party at my friend's house with her family and friends. By all accounts, I loved this friend and enjoyed hanging out with her. However, my boyfriend was back in Minnesota hanging out at a party with his friends—who had also become my friends. I felt so disoriented being away from him, even though I was back in a setting I was familiar with. It felt awful that we were both having good times—without each other. At the time, I couldn't quite process this, but now in hindsight, I realize this was a clear sign I'd lost my own identity in my relationship.

In comparison, today, my husband and I can easily have a great time together or independently, without anyone feeling left out. My husband enjoys playing baseball, and I enjoy sitting around reading books. We don't expect the other person to like what we like, and we don't always have to do something together. We are our own people first, and we get to choose to spend our time together. That is very different from depending on another person to fill a space you cannot fill on your own.

While your first instance of losing yourself is likely to be to a romantic relationship, there are other places you can lose yourself along the way. Becoming a first-time parent or entering a really intense job situation are a couple of other situations where you may be so consumed with the needs of others, you forget to tend to your own. Ultimately, this leads to unhealthy relationships and burnout.

So, how can you identify if you've lost yourself along your journey, whether this is due to a relationship or something else? Here are some behaviors to look out for.

1. An *emotional response* to an event where you're by yourself. For example, I was emotional over being at a party—that by all indications I should have been having fun at—simply because I wasn't with my boyfriend at the time.
2. *Lack of alone time* or discomfort with alone time. If you find you're never spending time by yourself, doing things that you want to do, this could be a signal you've lost yourself.
3. *Deferring to others' preferences* all the time. Sure, it's a kind gesture when someone comes to visit you from out of town to defer to their preferred restaurant for dinner. However, if you find yourself saying something like, "Well, what do you want?" every time your friend or partner asks you what you'd like for dinner, you might be losing sight of what you truly enjoy.

4. *Numbing behaviors*—like eating when you're not hungry, drinking frequently just because there doesn't seem to be anything better to do, or scrolling social media the whole night. We numb because we're uncomfortable and we want a distraction. That discomfort could be with your own codependency or lack of motivation and direction of your own.

If one or more of these is true, how might you find yourself again? Here are the ways in which I found my way back to myself.

FINDING AND REMEMBERING YOUR PURPOSE.

At this stage of my career and at thirty-four years old, I can articulate my purpose far better than I could when I left home at sixteen. Now I have a strong spiritual connection with the guiding lights in my life. I also have a life that includes a family to care for and a well-defined career path. Both aspects of my life are core components of my purpose for waking up every day.

At sixteen, I didn't have a solid foundation of an independent life just yet, but I did have a gut sense of what was the next right step in my path, and that came from my sense of purpose. In my worldview, that purpose is given to me as part of my faith in God, and the purpose I could articulate at that time was to simply make the world a better place. This led me to pursue skills that would help me on that journey and also to seek out opportunities to connect with and serve others. At thirty-four, I now know I specifically want to make: 1) healthcare and higher learning better for people living with chronic illnesses and disabilities, and 2) the workplace better for women who want to raise families while they have careers in science. Every day, waking up to care for my family and work on projects in my field of expertise are steps toward making that impact.

What I want you to notice is that no matter how far along you are in building your foundation of independent life, you can still have purpose. Someday, you may clearly be able to articulate a macro-purpose for your life, but it's OK if today you can only see a micro-purpose. Something as simple as reaching out to someone you know has been going through a tough time is part of having a greater purpose.

Having a sense of your purpose is important because it gives you the ability to aim at something positive. Think about shooting a bow and arrow. If you have a target, you will naturally turn toward and aim at that target. If you don't have anything to aim at, you have no idea where to point your bow, meaning you take a shot that wastes your time and your available resource of arrows.

Losing yourself is the equivalent to giving away your target. Without a target to aim at, you'll likely do things that waste your time and resources without making you happy. Part of finding yourself is knowing and claiming your target. With a target, you're going to take steps that feel in sync with who you are and what you enjoy.

If you don't yet know your targeted purpose, start by thinking about activities that light you up with joy. Think about skills that might be helpful to have for bigger goals you have in your life. Ponder on those big dreams and goals, even if they seem far out of reach right now. These are all lifelines toward your purpose.

STICK TO LIFE-GIVING HABITS.

When you're in a period where you feel lost, you also need to find your solid ground. The challenge is that when you are in a rough patch, it's also easy to find comfort in habits that do not nourish your mind or soul. Numbing behaviors like binge-watching Netflix, drinking too much, or overeating may make you feel better in the moment. However, afterward, you feel just as empty and lost as before. You only distracted and numbed yourself from it. To find yourself again, you need time where you're present, even when it hurts like heck, to process your feelings.

For me, there were two habits I clung to when I was going through the season following my breakup from my previous boyfriend and trying to refind myself: studying at the coffee shop and watching *Meet the Press*. Every day I would spend time at the coffee shop across the street from my apartment. The best way I can describe that place is to imagine the old TV show *Cheers*, except with espresso instead of beer. This habit was extremely important to regaining my sense of self because it made me feel less alone, and it kept me accountable to my goals of continuing to do well in my classes—all connected back to my purpose.

My other habit was to watch *Meet the Press* every Sunday. For a political science major, it made sense that I would like, and still do like, a political analysis show. The real purpose behind this habit, though, was that Sunday was hard—perhaps the hardest day of the week for me in the aftermath of my breakup—because it was a day that my boyfriend and I would usually spend together. Now Sundays were just lonely and empty.

So, I made it my Sunday habit to wake up just before 8 a.m., make myself something to eat and a nice cup of hot tea, then crawl back into bed and have my breakfast while I watched the show. It gave me something to look forward to each Sunday, even if it was the hardest day of the week. It also got me into a routine of getting up for the day instead of moping around all day in bed. And it was dedicated to a nerdy activity that I alone enjoyed independent of anyone else.

In another instance, early on as a first-time mother, I remember also feeling a bit like I'd lost myself. It was not in the same awful, heartbreaking way as a breakup, but rather that my body had been given to another person for nine months and still very much felt that way in the early newborn days. In that season, my husband would hang out with our son a few days a week so I could go to the gym for a workout. This separate activity just to myself that I enjoyed was life-giving and helped me reclaim my sense of self.

Be aware of both the habits that are harmful and the ones that make you whole. Make sure you find soul-nourishing habits as a way back to yourself. These might be things that you already did and are now renewing your commitment to, or they could be something new. Focus on finding one habit that can help you feel personal joy—like watching *Meet the Press* for me—and one that can keep you on track with your goals—like the coffee shop study sessions were for me.

REFLECTION PROMPTS:

- Where have you felt like you have lost track of yourself, now or in the past? What life events have triggered this—a relationship, a new phase of life like parenting, or something else?
- Which of the four signals (emotional responses to being alone, lack of or discomfort with alone time, deferring to others' preferences all the time, or numbing behaviors) do you notice happening when you feel lost?
- Can you specifically state what you feel like your life purpose is currently? Remember, you don't need to have a be-all and end-all statement of your life purpose; just focus on what tugs on your heart as important where you're at.
- What habits have you engaged with that really feel soul-nourishing for you?
- What are some new healthy habits that you'd want to explore? Consider one that is purely joyful and one that keeps you on track with your goals.

"Make sure you find soul-nourishing habits as a way back to yourself."

ANTIDOTES FOR

Impostor Syndrome

Have you ever wondered, "What if they find out I'm really not qualified for this?" Maybe you've even wondered this when your rational brain knows that you're more than qualified. This cognitive dissonance about whether you truly belong in a space or are a fraud is called impostor syndrome.

About a year and a half after moving to Minnesota, I enrolled in an undergraduate program at the University of Minnesota. In 2011, after completing my degree, I was hired as an administrative assistant in a research lab at a large healthcare organization. It wasn't long into my time in this position that my focus on graduate school began to crystallize. In order to accelerate my growth and make a greater impact, I would need to pursue a master's degree. So, in the summer of 2012, I began a master's in public health (MPH) program. In this same summer, I also happened to be a newlywed and seven months pregnant. To say I didn't look like the majority of my MPH cohort or my coworkers would be a massive understatement. My impostor syndrome showed up as "who do you think you are, going to grad school, working full time, and raising a family?" Quite truthfully, many people had both implicitly and explicitly told me what I was attempting was impossible. Even further, despite excellent mentorship in general, I didn't have anyone around me to look up to specifically as a role model for the path I was taking.

At the time, the fact that I didn't have a role model for the achiever scientist mama dealing with chronic illness seemed strange to me. I often thought to myself, "I can't be the only one to do this." It certainly increased my feelings of impostor syndrome, because if you look around and cannot see anyone like you doing what you're hoping to do after graduation, it is very easy to assume you truly don't belong in the room—the people around you are the experts, and you're the phony trying to play a part.

I wasn't imagining things either. Finding a woman who was married, with kids, and also living with a chronic illness at a high level of leadership was kind of like looking for a needle in a haystack. The National Institutes of Health (NIH) notes that even though in the past decade women earned nearly half of the science and engineering undergraduate and graduate degrees, less than 25 percent of those at the top rank in my field—full professors—are women.[1] Layer that with the fact that despite 20 percent of the US population living with some form of disability, only about 6 percent of graduates in science and engineering have disabilities.[2] A lack of role models has real consequences. When you don't have someone like you to help you navigate your professional spaces, you miss out on being educated in the rules of the game. These rules, or the *hidden curriculum*, are the "unspoken norms, values, and behaviors that exist within the learning environment."[3] Across several domains, extra support is needed to bring diverse trainees up to speed on how things work. These include training on how to withstand setbacks and develop a career with confidence.

Those were the facts I was facing that gave me impostor syndrome. If I don't see anyone around me who is like me, do I really belong here? However, everyone's impostor syndrome looks different. It could look like you're trucking along, hitting your goals in stride, and inside your head you're wondering how the heck this is working—you shouldn't be hitting this many good fortunes. It might also look like you're flunking your hardest class and barely hanging on to your part-time job because you're preoccupied trying to salvage your grade. As a result, you're pretty sure your advisor is going to call you in to their office and tell you your admission to the program was a complete mistake. *No matter the precise aspects of your impostor syndrome, it says: you are faking and someone will find out.*

I think one of the things we universally believe when we are the up-and-comer in sports, school, career, parenting, or anything else is that those more senior than us have it all figured out. Not only that, but they also got to where they are now flawlessly. However, if you peel back the curtain, I guarantee you, your mentors' successes are built on top of failure after failure after failure. More so, your mentors still have days where they wonder how they'll make it all work.

Right now, even as I mentor and teach others, some days I still worry about how I will take care of myself and show up strong enough for everyone around me—my family, my friends, and my colleagues—especially when my body is not cooperating as I'd like it to. Right now, even though it is not nearly as present as it was earlier in my life, I still get small gut-checks of impostor syndrome.

Here's what I want you to remember, though: *impostor syndrome thrives in the dark*. In hiding your impostor syndrome, it's just you who is experiencing this feeling. In the light, though, you realize *everyone is feeling or has felt this feeling*. Just to give you some examples, here's what some of my students and mentees have told me over the past few years.

1. Everyone around me is taking more advanced classes and has a higher grade point average than me, yet I'm still here.
2. Everyone in my lab has their dissertation figured out, and I'm still not sure I'm even in the right area.
3. I'm afraid that at some point, the program is going to figure out I don't fit in and they made a mistake selecting me.
4. I'm afraid no matter how hard I try, my test scores will keep me from getting into medical school and becoming a doctor.
5. Everyone is pushing me toward this one field, but I know based on my experience now, I won't be fulfilled long term. I am afraid if I ask about this, they'll wonder why they wasted their time training me.

Do you see yourself in any of those statements? Here's an interesting observation about these fears. They, on one hand, highlight that you're not alone in your impostor syndrome. On the other hand, they also highlight that everyone is on their own journey. You're not flying solo, but everyone's definition of "figuring it out" is going to look a little bit different. If you let noticing others' journeys turn into comparison, this can also amplify your feelings of impostor syndrome.

I will say, though, in my own impostor syndrome, I did find it helpful to understand that even if it looked different for other people, they too thought someone was going to figure out they didn't belong for one reason or another. It also was critically important that I trusted myself—that my life and career dreams were possible and that I had the qualifications and drive to pursue them, regardless of external circumstances.

Nowadays, I can hope that there is another early-career person out there who wants a family, a degree, and a job simultaneously who can use the journey I took as a light for the path that they are on. I hope by sharing my stories, they can see that in no way was this dream forged in perfection. Instead, it was messy, and there were failures. Yet, despite this, I kept going. I kept trusting that I was learning, growing, and doing my best. I kept trusting that even when I felt like I was faking it until I made it, I did belong where I was.

Here are some of the strategies I used to gain this confidence.

KNOW THYSELF THROUGH ASSESSMENT.

Depending on your upbringing and spiritual perspectives, you may believe each of us is uniquely created by a supreme being, the result of incredible odds to somehow be a tiny speck in time and cosmos, or something in between. Regardless, we each are individual in our DNA makeup and the environment in which we developed. Therefore, it is critically important to know that you may be comparing your skills and your journey to a person who is absolutely nothing like you. You need to know the facets of your unique self, or else you begin to think you don't stack up to someone who has a completely different set of DNA and life circumstances.

For example, maybe you're naturally on the reserved side in social situations and you feel like an impostor next to the public speaker in your class who seems to have been born ready for a microphone. Maybe you're great at seeing the big picture and terrible at figuring out the details, but you feel most inferior next to the person with a ten-bullet-point list. If you think of only another person's strengths and how you fall short of their strengths, you will have a high likelihood of feeling like an impostor. If, instead, you think about the other person's strengths as unique to them, and then think about the strengths that are specific to you, you can see how each person makes a different contribution to the world.

For example, my strengths are being vision oriented, a strategic thinker, unfailingly positive, and a teacher/mentor to others. The strengths of one of my colleagues are being detail oriented, service oriented, and a deep, introverted thinker. I build and design programs, bring on team members who can help us achieve our goals, and find funding for projects. My colleague, on the other hand, is crucial to ensuring that projects get carried out. She manages the fine details of making sure everything is in place to execute the plan. She catches critical errors on funding applications I miss when looking at the big picture. I don't feel inferior to her, nor she to me. Rather, the team fails without both people with unique strengths.

In addition to seeing the different contributions of everyone, examining my own strengths and weaknesses also helps me better take care of myself so I can take care of others. For example, I give a great deal of my attention to others' needs through activities like teaching and mentoring. I also know that my best creative work happens internally with intuition, rather than out-loud brainstorming. I love systems and structure that help me act on my many goals. While I have become much better at going with the flow, particularly when it comes to spending quality time with my family, I still feel my best when most of my week is clearly planned out and I have a daily checklist.

Knowing this about myself helps me understand things about myself—for example, when I am feeling particularly tired, it is often because I have spent a great deal of time extroverting. When I am feeling particularly unproductive or life is chaotic, I probably haven't spent enough time in planning mode. I know what it takes to make my unique contribution to the world and how to appreciate the strengths of others.

You can reflect on your own strengths by reflecting on the

following.

- When do you feel your most energized? If you're feeling low on energy, what can you do to bring yourself out of a funk?
- What are you uniquely good at helping others do or learn?
- How do you make your best decisions? Conversely, when you've made poor decisions, what were the circumstances that drove you to them?
- Are you more at ease going with the flow or when you structure your days? How can you maximize the best of both worlds when life gives you both?
- Think of someone who is very different from you—what are their strengths, and what do you admire about them?

Looking at your reflections here, what would you name as your key three strengths? How do you use them in the world to make it a better place?

KNOW THYSELF THROUGH REFLECTION.

Knowing yourself generally through assessment is foundational. However, regular attention is needed to build upon this foundation. Specifically, you need to develop a strong, regularly visited relationship with yourself to tame impostor syndrome. I have observed many who do not actively think about or pay careful attention to cultivating a relationship with themselves. Because of this, they spend most of their time in reaction mode, rather than reflecting on past and future situations to maximize their potential and growth.

Spending time with and on yourself isn't self-centered or selfish. If you do not know yourself well, you will not be able to help others from a grounded place. When you have a regular practice of reflection, it is much easier to put impostor syndrome in its proper place. If all your time is filled with other peoples' voices and opinions, you are not going to be able to fully pay attention to *your* truth.

The reason a lot of people don't spend this critical time reflecting and cultivating a relationship with themselves is that it requires you to sit with your own thoughts. Turns out, for most humans, sitting alone in quiet with your thoughts is kind of scary. I do not mean sitting alone in a quiet room scrolling social media or the news. Nor do I mean sitting at a coffee shop reading the latest book. Anything that requires consumption of information ultimately distracts you from tuning in to the thoughts that are roaming around in your head.

Self-reflection comes through activities like sitting silently, meditating, or reflecting with calming music. For others, it may be best done walking in nature. Ultimately, I cannot tell you about your best method for self-reflection. However, I can share what has worked for me and hope that it gives you some decent ideas about where to start.

I just close my eyes and meditate and make space for my thoughts. No, just kidding. I feel calm enough to do this on 0.5 percent of days.

For me, I have found the best method of cultivating a relationship with myself, and therefore falling less often into impostor syndrome, is through journaling. Some people I have worked with worry that someone is going to read their journal—in some cases just because they don't want anyone to know what's going on in their head, and in other cases for their actual safety and well-being. If that is something you struggle with, writing something down on a separate sheet of paper that you can burn or shred or flush down the toilet may be a better option for you.

My journaling is a space to put down on paper messy thoughts and emotions that are circling in my head. It serves as a brain dump to help me get to know myself, rather than acting in a reactionary mode all the time. As I do this, I also examine whether there are certain thoughts or emotions that are pent up and possibly holding me back. In doing so, I recognize that I, like any human, think a lot of unhelpful thoughts. I need to see them written out to reframe them.

For example, if you receive a rejection for a position from a job interview, you might think, "I knew I wasn't good enough; they saw right through me." That thought makes you feel like an impostor—and makes you less likely to try again for the next job interview. In the face of rejection, you could instead think, "That position just wasn't the best fit for me or the organization. I need to find something more aligned with my energy and goals." That thought motivates you to search for something that is better for you anyway. Instead of an impostor hiding, you're confident that your skills are great for something that just hasn't come along yet.

A method that you can use to reflect on your own thoughts is to select a goal that you're working toward or want to work toward but haven't gotten the courage to do so yet. Sit down with a paper, pen, and timer set for ten minutes. Start the timer and write down every thought that comes to mind about this goal until the timer goes off. Write freely until the timer stops. Then look at what you've written down. Realistically consider which thoughts are helpful versus unhelpful to pursuing your goal.

Of the thoughts that are unhelpful, are there ways that you can reframe them to be neutral or positive? For example, your goal might be to achieve a 3.5 GPA this semester. An unhelpful thought you may have written down is, "I am always behind on classwork. Because I am so unorganized, I can't achieve the GPA I want." To reframe this positively, you might instead say, "I am working on my organization skills. By paying attention to these little details, I am getting closer to my desired GPA." Or, more neutrally, "Last semester, I turned in assignments late. This semester, I am turning them in on time." When you read those sentences, notice how toggling between different thoughts about the same set of circumstances can produce radically different feelings. Which thought makes you feel more energized and ready to keep tackling your goal?

Do this exercise regularly, at least once every couple of weeks, or anytime you feel your impostor syndrome creeping up. Unhelpful thoughts are kind of like cobwebs in our brain. They accumulate and block our ability to see things we're working on clearly. This journaling exercise can clear out those cobwebs and help you realign yourself with your goals.

REFLECTION PROMPTS:

- What do I currently know about myself and my strengths?
- How do I bring these strengths to the world without falling into a comparison trap with others?
- What person or ideal am I comparing myself to when I experience feelings of impostor syndrome?
- How often am I spending time reflecting on unhelpful thoughts?
- What thoughts are driving my emotions and actions? Do I like where they're driving me, or would I like to think different, more useful thoughts?

"If you do not know yourself well, you will not be able to help others from a grounded place."

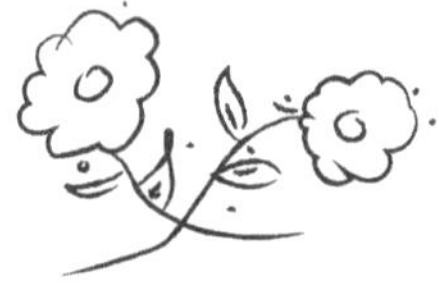

PART II

ANTIDOTES FOR

Facing the Pressure of Deadlines

There aren't very many paths you can take in life that don't require you to meet some sort of deadline. If you are a college student, you'll face deadlines for midterms and final papers. If you become a salesperson, you'll face deadlines to make sales goals to get a bonus. As an academic, I face deadlines for grant funding and manuscript revisions. As a parent, I face deadlines to sign my oldest up for the next hockey training camp and to get the school supplies ordered before the first day of school. Whatever path you choose, deadlines are a nonnegotiable aspect of life.

I learned about deadlines at a very young age, and in hindsight, I can see how this learning served me well in my early adulthood. My first recollection of exposure to deadlines was around age seven, sitting on the floor of my mother's office at Region 9 Education Service Center in Wichita Falls, Texas. My mom was an educator and an education administrator, and the programs she ran required grant funding. For those of you unfamiliar with grant funding, it is a method by which you propose an idea to an agency that awards funds to the best proposal(s) for those ideas. Sometimes these granting agencies are governmental, and other times they are nonprofit, philanthropic, or industry related. No matter what kind of agency you are submitting a grant to, they have a deadline by which you need to turn in your application.

One of my most vivid memories at seven years old was watching how meeting a deadline unfolded. At the time, electronic submissions weren't a thing; all submissions were in the form of paper copies. This meant you could buy yourself some time by turning in your grant proposal (usually multiple large boxes of papers) by hand, instead of trusting the postal mail with it. If you sent your grant proposal paper copies by postal mail, you had to send it out a few days in advance, so that it would be stamped as received at the granting agency by the due date. However, if you decided to drive the paper copies to the agency, you could bring them in the day of the deadline and have them stamped *received* right in front of you. Given that this extended your work time before turning in the grant, my mom often chose this second, road-trip-required option (and I don't blame her one bit). As such, my life included many car trips to the granting agencies, primarily based in Austin, Texas, to physically turn grants in by their deadline. Austin was a five-hour trip from home. That's dedication.

Sometimes when Mom was working on a deadline, she would take me home first after school, cook supper for us, and then go back to her office alone to continue working (this was long before the days of laptop computers or remote work). Other times, when both she and Dad, who ran a nonprofit business, were simultaneously working on deadlines, she would get me McDonald's for dinner and we would stay at her office well into the evening while she worked. On these evenings, my main understanding of the time that passed was not by the clock, but rather by whether we left before the janitor came by to empty our trash and talk to us.

While she worked, I would explore her office library, which was vast and filled with books on every topic you could imagine. I would take my book of choice and sit on the floor, often for hours. I would work through the book, sometimes teaching my dolls as if I were a teacher just like her. I always sat facing her desk. She would write, alternating between the early version of a personal computer and a digital typewriter.

These experiences didn't seem peculiar to me at the time, and I am grateful for the leadership above her that saw education as all-encompassing, including bring-your-kid-to-work-after-school education. However, now when I look back on it, I realize I had an exceptional childhood. Not because of toys, a particularly expansive house, or a ton of money. No, my childhood was exceptional because of deadlines. My parents role-modeled how to meet deadlines to the best of your abilities with fervor and grace. I also learned that people think things get accomplished through motivation and inspiration, but no, friend, things get accomplished through the structure given by deadlines.

This role modeling set me on a path for a very strong start in my early career. When I transitioned from my undergraduate education into the workplace, my exposure to deadlines grew exponentially. My first job out of undergraduate was as an administrative assistant in the research unit where I am a lead researcher and professor. As an administrative assistant, you are handed a stack of deadlines to manage for yourself and others. I was required to schedule meetings for people within a short time frame. I was also expected to understand timelines for our team's grant submissions and progress reports and coordinate timelines to meet those deadlines.

Within my first year on the job, I became pregnant with our first child, Owen, while I simultaneously started graduate schoolwork. Now I had not one set of deadlines but three—work, school, and family—to oversee. In hindsight, thank *heavens* my mother role-modeled what being a good mom and meeting deadlines looked like, because I wouldn't have been as prepared for this challenge had she not. Here are some things I learned from her and that I found to be particularly helpful in facing deadlines in my very real, messy life.

DON'T WASTE SPARE TIME.

In the goal-setting lexicon, you will see advice that talks about focusing on what you want to accomplish for that day or block of hours and not truly stopping until it gets accomplished. For example, you might see someone say focus on getting your new kitchen backsplash up today. Focus on writing the introduction and methods sections of your academic paper this week. Focus on finishing reading five chapters in your psychology textbook this week. Collect all the background information you need before you close your computer for the day. I could go on, but you get the point.

Those are great aspirations, y'all. Fabulous. Here's the deal, though. *As a mom trying to manage a household, a career, and an ed-*

ucation, I learned that type of advice was a pipe dream. My life was never bound by me getting the discussion section written; it was bound by what time I had to drop what I was doing to read a bedtime story. My morning meditation was never bound by an aha moment. It was bound by what time I had to wake my son up to go to school. I always had the endgame in mind, such as finishing a grant or my dissertation. I just never knew how much of it I was going to get done when I sat down for a finite number of minutes. What I could control was using the time I had as productively as I could and picking right back up where I left off at the next opportunity.

What making this work looks like in my very real life is 1) having a list of important projects I am working on and their status, and 2) looking at my calendar for slivers of time.

When you create your list of your important projects, you need to note 1) the level of importance of this project for your current phase of growth, and 2) the project deadline. Ultimately, you should periodically evaluate what makes something a priority in your work, because as you become more successful, you will either be asked or want to do more things than you have time for in a single season of your life. For example, early in your career, you likely will be primarily working for someone who is creating your deadlines. This was certainly true for me early in my career when I was an administrative assistant and a graduate student. The deadlines that I had were ones assigned by others. As you get further along in your career, you begin to have more autonomy regarding what is important and how you want to prioritize your time. Now, as a lead researcher and assistant professor, more of the deadlines I have are imposed by myself to further my career to create positive impact in the world. Sure, I could forego a grant deadline this fall, but that would have serious negative implications for my career growth and ability to help others with my research.

Let's think about how this applies to your life. For simplicity in working through this antidote example, let's say you're starting out in your career, and you have a sales report due to your boss in one week. This is a highly important task. If you do not successfully get this report to your boss on time, they will be upset, and it will hurt your chances for promotion.

Looking at this task, you know you have plenty of time to complete the report in a single day. However, you know such uninterrupted, dedicated time isn't going to happen because you're the go-to person in the office for fast, reliable information-gathering. You get distracted multiple times in a day, and even when you have time blocked off in your day to work on your report due next week, people still may interrupt you. It's hard to reliably find time at home because you have a partner and young kids who you want to spend time with when you're together.

Knowing this background, you realize you need to find multiple opportunities to work on your report, such that inevitably getting sidetracked a few times won't seriously damage your ability to complete the task on time. This is where tiny time slivers become important and are often overlooked. It turns out, if you look at your upcoming week, you have lots of spare minutes, if you remind yourself to stay focused on the sales report. As such, in addition to blocking time on your calendar to get the report done, you also keep it pulled up in the background along with a sticky note about where you left off. That way, when you find some spare time during the day, you immediately start back on the report where you stopped earlier.

One of the biggest detriments to productivity or progress in our lives is saying, "I don't have enough time." You do. Full stop, you do. You may feel angry at me for saying that—for calling you out on it—but I swear you do. I know you do because I do too! I'm just as guilty, if I don't self-monitor, of using those twenty minutes in between my next appointment to scroll the news or peep at X (formerly Twitter) instead of using them to write that important email. It's not to say that there isn't a time and place for brain rest—every second of every day shouldn't be filled with work. There should be times for rest, relaxation, and leisure in there as well; I personally like to schedule these into my calendar too. Just don't waste all your slivers of spare time during the day zoning out or using numbing behaviors to avoid the thing you don't want to do. Try spending a couple of those slivers of downtime doing something that will move the needle forward.

It may help to go back a few chapters and look at your time tracking. If you were honest in that activity, you can identify where you do have time, even if it is ten minutes here or twenty minutes there. Think about it. How badly do you want it—this dream—whatever it is for you? What, if over a year's time, using a few slivers of extra minutes every day added up to finishing a grad school course that you have been convincing yourself you don't have time for? What if those extra minutes added up to starting and growing the business you keep dreaming about?

GIVE YOURSELF GRACE.

My mother's role-modeling taught me that meeting a big deadline is hard. It's hard because it pulls the life out of you and requires all your energy and focus to go to that single thing. But that single thing is not likely the be-all and end-all in your life. You have friends. You have a family. You may have a spouse. You may have kids. What my childhood taught me with my parents often on deadlines is that bringing your family along for the journey is OK too.

I look back on childhood so fondly. And yet so many moms who lived my mom's life today would be posting on social media about mom guilt. Maybe she had it. I don't know. She certainly never showed it. She just showed me what it looked like to be a badass lady, and that's what I remember. Your kids are going to remember what you taught them with your actions just as much, if not more, than your words. I can see the evidence that my oldest son knows in his spirit what it is like to chase a big goal in his hockey career because he watched me chase my goal of a doctoral degree for so long. If you don't neglect your loved ones while following your dreams, but instead bring them along for the ride, they will benefit from the experience as well. So please, when you're juggling a deadline and trying to also show up for your people, give yourself a little grace.

Please forgive yourself when meeting a deadline means you feed your kid a freezer meal or McDonald's for the fourth time this week. Don't do it all the time—feed them healthy things when you can. But I promise you, my kid is fine after surviving me doing two graduate degrees during his young life. I promise you fast food and a messy house were part of the equation sometimes. My point is, quit being so quick to judge yourself for the sacrifices you're making for your dreams. Deadlines are part of dreams, y'all. So give yourself permission to meet your deadline and pick up all the things that took a backseat after it's done. Once that deadline is met, make sure you rest, recover, and enjoy some free time before getting back to the work once again.

Deadlines are challenging, but you got this.

REFLECTION PROMPTS:

- How do you currently think about deadlines and approach them when they arise?
- Where are you losing momentum because you're thinking you must get something completed?
- Where could you find a few minutes each day to make progress toward your most important deadline?
- When have you been hard on yourself for letting something slide when you're working on a deadline? How might you show yourself grace instead?

"One of the biggest detriments to productivity or progress in our lives is saying, 'I don't have enough time.'"

ANTIDOTES FOR

When You Get Sidetracked

"I'm so behind," I thought, as I lit the metaphorical nighttime candle of continued work well past a reasonable bedtime hour. I kept myself awake with a late-night cup of tea, just a little bit more caffeine to get me through the last couple of hours of studying and working. I told myself this lie time and time again, as I sustained this ritual for a few years.

"If I could just lose five more pounds, directly from my midsection, of course, I'd be happier with my body," I said as I looked into the mirror for the umpteenth time that month. I restricted my caloric intake, ate more vegetables and fewer carbs, and did lose the few pounds, but in the end, I wasn't any happier with my body. My body had been fine the way it was.

"His perception of me matters," I told myself as I pushed myself to climb a career ladder that was a mirage in my head because nobody had ever climbed *this* exact climb before. "I should do x, y, and z to impress this person in the event that they have some bearing on my next steps."

These are all lies that I have told myself in the past. In hindsight I see that each sidetracked me away from things that ultimately matter, like my purpose, my family, and my well-being.

February of 2016 changed all that. It was the beginning of my second semester of the PhD program; I was also working full time as an analyst, and my oldest was three years old. It was a Thursday evening, and I was driving the hour and a half home from a class. It was a typical cold, slow drive on a February day, and I noticed some low pelvic pain. Within a day or two I was certain I had a urinary tract infection (UTI). I called the nurse line and was prescribed antibiotics over the phone. A few days later, I felt no different. In the back of my mind, I knew that the other two times I had UTIs, I was much better within the same time frame.

The lack of relief persisted, even after I took all my antibiotics. In fact, I continued to feel worse. This time, when I called the nurse line, I was advised to be seen in clinic. This doctor diagnosed my pain as pelvic inflammatory disease (PID). Honestly, I had never heard of PID until this moment but learned that it was an infection of one of the female reproductive organs. What I also learned was that as a married, monogamous woman, I was not at high risk for PID. I felt this was odd, but they assured me some people just had bad luck and got it anyway. I was given a strong antibiotic injection and sent home with two additional antibiotics for a ten-day course. This time, I did feel relief. Unfortunately, it lasted only a week. The pain showed up again like an unwanted solicitor at my front door.

I texted my friend and colleague who is a physician and asked, "Can PID return? I'm beginning to have pain again." She replied, "Not usually." At this point I felt like my body was betraying me, and I couldn't see an end in sight. I returned to the primary care clinic, and they were equally perplexed. PID didn't usually return, but it was their only good hypothesis. I needed a visit with a gynecologist to explore further reasons for my sudden, unrelenting pain. But getting an appointment with a specialist can often take months, which feels overwhelming when you're in continual pain. Thankfully, I had colleagues that could help expedite the process, but it wasn't immediate.

A week before my gynecology appointment, my husband insisted he take me to the emergency department (ED); I could barely walk because of the pain. At the ED, the team marveled at my perfect vitals, an indication of how healthy I was. Yet for some unknown reason, within the span of two months I could no longer function because of pelvic pain. I was able to receive some pain medication, which at least kept me comfortable while I waited for further consultation, but it was not a long-term solution. When my gynecology appointment came around, the physician examined me and said, "Really, I think you still have PID; we will send you home with some more antibiotics." I began to sob in his office. I had never felt so dejected in my life. My head was screaming, "This is NOT the right diagnosis," and yet all that would come out was tears.

Turns out most men are called to action when a perfectly composed woman dissolves into tears. He hustled to the Kleenex box and offered me some. Then he asked, "You're crying because you don't think this is going to work?"

I replied, "Yes, I don't think PID is what is going on with my body, and I don't want to be sent home alone to figure it out myself."

With this, he agreed to admit me to the hospital for a five-day course of IV antibiotics. I didn't love this option, but I reasoned at least I would be monitored 24/7 by a medical team. Four days into my planned five-day hospital stay, I had no improvement in my symptoms. I still needed medication at regular intervals to manage the unrelenting pain. On that fourth day, the female supervising physician who had been there at the time I was admitted came in to talk to me. She looked at me kindly and with a sense of solidarity said, "You knew giving you five more days of antibiotics inpatient wouldn't help, didn't you?" I nodded, confiding in her that I had assumed it wouldn't work, but it was the only good option on the table at the time if I didn't want to be sent home to manage alone. And so, the next day I was sent for exploratory surgery.

Yet, even when they cut me open, they could find *absolutely nothing* to indicate why I was in miserable pain.

Admittedly desperate to claw my way out of pain following the hospitalization and surgery, I began to put the pieces of the puzzle together myself. I had suspected much of the time that there was a good chance it was my bladder causing the problem. I reasoned that I'd had a finicky bladder my whole life, but it was still bizarre because this tiny little organ had never caused me any pain, much less *severe pain*. Yet, with no gynecologic or gastrointestinal reason for my pain, my bladder seemed to be the most likely culprit. Why was it revolting now?

It turns out, bodies charge interest on the care you withhold from them, and so I think the limited sleep and maximum caffeine intake was finally catching up to me. My body could no longer withstand such treatment and needed time to heal. As I tried to figure out what was happening with my body, I learned that there is a well-established correlation between stress and symptom flares in many chronic conditions, although the exact mechanisms are typically unclear. For example, in a survey of patients with lupus, increases in daily stress appeared to increase patient-reported increased symptoms within the next two days.[1] Over the coming months, I would be diagnosed with interstitial cystitis or bladder pain syndrome (IC/BPS), another condition in which stress is commonly associated with symptom flares.[2] With this, I would begin medications and nonpharmacologic treatment strategies.

IC/BPS was my first chronic condition diagnosis in adulthood, but my fourth overall. Its arrival not only changed my medications and lifestyle, but also changed where I put my energy. Some key components to ensure I stay functioning with IC/BPS are regular nights of seven-plus hours of sleep, exercise at least five days per week, and time reserved for just relaxation. It also requires that I take my medications multiple times a day and attend treatment appointments at least monthly. When I consider the list of activities that I must do to stay well, plus the commitment I have to my family and the obligations I have to my career, I don't have time to waste on things that really don't matter anymore. So, here is how that reframed those lies I told myself years ago.

"I am not behind in anything, nor am I ahead in anything." I am simply where I am. All things will get done, and if they don't, they probably weren't that important anyway. I will make progress daily toward my goals, but not to the point it sacrifices time with the ones I love or the sleep that I need to function.

"Weight does not define anything other than my relationship with the gravitational pull of the earth; strength is what actually matters." I focus now entirely on gaining strength and loving myself when I look in the mirror.

"I have zero bearing on anyone's thoughts other than my own." I cannot control or even influence another person's perception of me. I can only control how I live and move authentically through the world. If that is out of sync with someone else's ideal, so what?

You may not have a life-altering diagnosis to shift your perspective on what truly matters. If you don't, it's still worthwhile to consider if what you're focusing on is important to your overall life's purpose and goals. Here are some antidotes for when you find yourself focusing on problems that distract you from the more important things in your life.

KNOW YOUR PILLARS.

Imagine yourself in a scenario like this one. You are working on a project, and you receive an email from a superior stating they found some critical problems with the work that has been done and it needs to be remedied. Rather than moving immediately into fixing the problem, your brain flies into panic thinking like, "Oh my gosh, they're going to think I do sloppy work," or "I can't believe I made such a careless mistake; how mortifying." You spend an hour or more in distress and feeling very upset. Ultimately, you have not made a single edit to the work yet. Not to mention, you probably had other things on your to-do list that have now been neglected as well.

Now, can you imagine a situation where you receive the same information via email, and instead of letting your brain roam around unmanaged, you take the feedback, edit the work, and turn the edits around before the day is over? Not only do you learn something, but you also get on with fixing the problem and don't sidetrack your day or mood. Maybe you need a little time to decompress by sharing with a coworker, but you do this in a brief and healthy way and then get on with the edits. The point being, you don't let the emotions of it all sidetrack you from getting things done.

A key strategy for successfully making this mental pivot is to have clear-cut definitions of what is important to you and boundaries around what you will and will not give your attention to. I call the things in my life that are fundamentally important my "pillars." If pillars fall, a structure crumbles. My pillars include activities like sleep, exercise, taking my medications, and paying attention to my family and goals. When I have my intentions and priorities clearly aligned such that my pillars are maintained, I am far less likely to get pulled into a negative spiral of thinking about any given situation that arises day to day.

Defining your pillars takes some work. You and only you can decide what activities, when neglected, leave you burnt out, sick, sad, or aimless. Some aspects of your life to consider are your physical, emotional, social, spiritual, aspirational, financial, or environmental needs. Once you define your goals and activities in these domains that require your daily or near-daily attention, you will likely realize there aren't very many minutes left in the day to get sidetracked by things that don't matter.

Y'all, no one's family is going to say when you are gone: "Well, at least she answered that email last night." They are going to remember you by what impact you made on their lives and the world. Your kids are going to remember that you tucked them into bed, and when you were not there tucking them into bed, it was because you needed to help other people in the world. Likewise, your partner is going to remember your date nights and the laughter.

As you define your own pillars, you may find yourself fearful of what happens when you need to enact a boundary to preserve a pillar. A good example of this is what happens when an email comes in with an urgent request while you're on vacation. If your pillars are to give adequate time to yourself for rest and for connection with your family, you would need to not check email during your vacation. Doing so would mean enabling the out-of-office notification on your email and you not seeing any of your emails until your return. Checking your email, seeing the request, and responding to it would sidetrack you from your pillars of rest and family. Yet, the idea of not seeing or responding to the request may make some overachievers' skin crawl.

Before you're ready to write this antidote off, try a new perspective first. Regardless of whether you work within a company or are an entrepreneur, people pay you for quality work. Not taking time to refresh will eventually diminish the quality of work you're doing. People don't want to pay full price for work you put 50 percent of your energy into. Give yourself permission to try taking this scary step of setting boundaries to protect your pillars with lots of upfront communication about when you'll be away and when you'll be back. If it still feels scary, you can experiment with doing this for a very short period, like a long weekend versus an extended vacation. Then pay attention to your ability to engage more fully after taking a true break.

PACE YOURSELF.

I think one of the easiest ways to get sidetracked is when you're moving so fast in life that you don't even notice you're off course. This might look like having goals but being so busy you haven't looked at them in more than a week. It also might look like having a to-do list that is so long, you end it every day with multiple undone tasks. Maybe it looks like exhaustion and feeling like you're constantly behind.

In today's world, a full calendar is glorified, but I don't know if anyone has paid attention to the downstream harms of such practice. I certainly didn't pay attention or buy into this prior to my earth-shaking IC/BPS diagnosis. It wasn't until I was on medical leave, doing a whole lot of nothing, that I realized how hard I had pushed myself consistently for so long.

Here's the thing. I *love* pushing myself. I'm the weirdo who wants to do the feel-like-you-might-die workout every day. This talent has always served me well because "hard" work and drive are glorified in this outcome-driven world. For some people this internal motivation and optimism is inherent, and for others they need to work on it. I personally have always been someone who can easily access my own intrinsic motivation. I also know folks who must spend a lot of mental energy in finding that motivation. I can convince myself to keep going at any cost. This can be a strength, but when it's overused, it's a liability to your happiness, your goals, and your health.

The antithesis to a tired, sidetracked person is a rested, intentional person. Do not fuel your late-night productivity binges on caffeine and lies of "If you just get through this last section, you'll be better off." No, you won't be better off. You will just be tired. And tomorrow, you will fuel yet another lie on another pot of coffee and trudge your way through it. On a rare occasion, you may need to make such heroic effort. But if you are doing this as a regular ritual, your pace is unsustainable. It is either unsustainable for your body, unsustainable for your spirit, or unsustainable for your loved ones. Worst of all, it may be unsustainable for all three.

Rested intentionality will look different for everyone, but for me it requires my morning routine and planned rest. I spend the first hour of my day reflecting and planning. I have a specific planning process I use during this time. First, at the beginning of the month, I reflect on the month's priorities, including upcoming deadlines and family activities. At the beginning of each week, I allocate weekly to-dos based upon the month's look-ahead. Then, I reflect on when I have concentrated work time without meetings available for writing and other concentrated tasks. Finally, at the beginning of each day, I reflect on the previous day, review meeting times for the day, and outline my to-do list. By planning and reflecting regularly, I can very easily spot when I have gotten sidetracked and what I need to do to get back on track. *You can use this process with the planning template on my website,* **www.kaseyboehmer.com**, *for free.*

When it comes to rest, I spend a good portion of my weekends resting. I sleep at least seven hours a night, and I schedule time off and self-care activities. These hard stops in life provide space for my body to recover and my brain to reset, both also foundational for noticing when I am off path.

Practice pace. Practice letting go of getting ahead. Practice marking your bedtime hour and honoring it. Practice not working until the last minute before you go to bed and, instead, talking with your friends or family, reading, watching a show or movie, playing a game, anything that takes you out of the mindset of working. I say practice because these actions will likely not come naturally. We tend to overwork, especially if we enjoy our jobs or the goals we're pursuing. Working more can increase our job satisfaction, but this comes with a cost of decreasing mental health[3] and physical health, particularly if the method by which you overwork is forgoing things like physical activity and sleep. Practice will not make you perfect, but it will make you better. Find a pace that moves you forward, protects your body, and makes sure you have your priorities at the forefront.

REFLECTION PROMPTS:

- What are some of the lies you've told yourself that don't serve your whole well-being?
- What are some small things you've spent time on recently that really won't matter in your long-term future?
- Have you experienced a period where your perspective changed regarding what is important in your life? If so, how did your perspective change from then to now?
- When you honestly think about the pace you're currently moving at, do you think it's sustainable? If yes, how do you know? If no, what needs to change?
- What do you know are your pillars to your overall well-being? What, if any, areas do you think you may need to better consider in terms of defining your pillars and what boundaries are required to protect those pillars?

RESOURCES:

Calendar planning template available at **www.kaseyboehmer.com.**

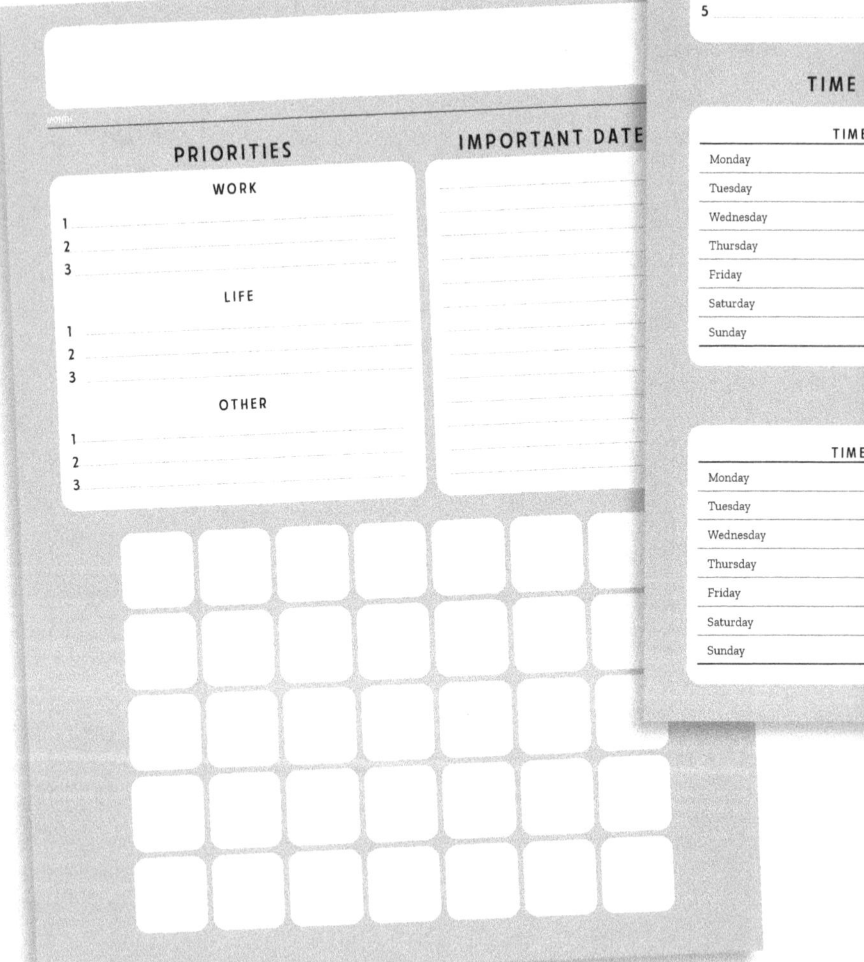

-DO LIST

6
7
8
9
10

VAILABLE FOR TO-D

TASK

FE EVENTS

E

TODAY'S DATE

TASKS

1
2
3
4
5

6
7
8
9
10

6 a.m.
7 a.m.
8 a.m.
9 a.m.
10 a.m.
11 a.m.
12 p.m.
1 p.m.

2 p.m.
3 p.m.
4 p.m.
5 p.m.
6 p.m.
7 p.m.
8 p.m.
9 p.m.

"The antithesis to a tired, sidetracked person is a rested, intentional person."

ANTIDOTES FOR

Naysayers

People looked at me a little bit strangely when I began my master's degree. One day in late December of 2011, I received an email telling me I had been accepted into the University of Minnesota's master of public health (MPH) program. The very next day, I received a positive pregnancy test. If I accepted my invitation to start my MPH, I would start the program the same summer I was due to deliver our first child. I also intended to continue working full time and thankfully had the support of my work unit to flex my hours as needed to accommodate coursework. No one told me I couldn't do it—but their looks didn't hide their skepticism.

Ultimately, I accepted the program invitation and delivered a healthy baby boy in the summer of 2012. I completed my MPH in two years on the standard, not extended, timeline. I graduated shortly before Owen turned two years old. At the completion of my MPH, I decided I wanted to continue graduate school and apply to get a PhD. When I shared my dreams this time around, looks turned into words. Many people were very quick to say my goal was impossible. I call these folks the naysayers; these are the people who are skeptical or cynical about what you want to accomplish. In some cases, naysayers flat out tell you that what you want to do is impossible.

At the time of preparing my application for a PhD, I met with numerous senior colleagues who very clearly told me that despite pulling it off with my MPH, completing a PhD while working full time with a family was just not a doable endeavor. Some said PhDs were designed to be full-time pursuits on their own without any paid work added on top. That didn't sit well with me, because even with a stipend, I couldn't contribute enough to our budget for a mortgage and day care without working. Others said that maybe I could pull off working while pursuing the PhD, but it would be at such a detriment to my family they'd barely know me. Those are some heavy words, and I did feel a tinge of hurt. I am grateful for my family and my primary mentor's support as I forged ahead through the cacophony of disbelief and disapproval.

In my heart of hearts, I knew I deeply wanted to get my PhD. I could not accomplish my goals in my career—to fund and carry out research that was driven by its importance to me—without that doctoral degree. I also knew in my heart of hearts that it could be done because my mom was my shining example. While she never went on to pursue a PhD, she did go back to complete a bachelor's degree and a master's degree as a mom. In my mind, anything my mom fundamentally believed could be done got done. She always said, "The time will pass anyway," which meant that the days, weeks, and years were going to move forward regardless of what you did with them. You might as well do something that is important to you while they pass. That's a legacy I wanted to leave for my family too—dedication to something that matters and the patience and persistence to see a goal to fruition.

So, after yet another conversation in which I was told I couldn't make this work, I strapped on my running shoes, cranked up Katy Perry's "Roar" in my headphones, and ran all the frustration out. I left it all on the pavement. No one was going to do this for me, and the naysayers were going to be there whether I went after it or not. I finished my run, and I started my PhD applications.

Months later after my defiant decision, I was accepted into the University of Minnesota's School of Nursing PhD program. I chose to go full time, juggling work and mom life yet again. My first semester, I took five courses. Let's just say that was probably outlandish; I am comfortable admitting that. And the physical toll that it took on my body, as evidenced by our discussion in the last chapter, was high. Eventually, though, I found a rhythm that did work for me, my body, my career, and my family. When I found that rhythm, it felt *good*. I was living out my dreams, and there is nothing as satisfying as seeing progress and growth toward big dreams—especially when the naysayers are watching from the sidelines.

Fast-forward to May of 2018. I donned a cap and gown and

walked across the stage at Northrop Auditorium to be hooded as Dr. Kasey Boehmer. Owen was now five years old. He sat in the audience with my parents and my husband. When I exited the stage, he ran through the aisle of the auditorium to catch me on the way to my seat. He gave me the biggest hug in the whole wide world, and said with tears in his eyes, "Mom, I'm so proud of you!" As I walked back to my seat, now with tears in my own eyes, I soaked in the feeling of accomplishment. No naysayer could ever take away the work I'd put in, but more importantly, no naysayer could have predicted that rather than my dreams being a detriment to my family, they'd been a blessing. Turns out, I gave birth to a goal-getter.

What my experience has shown me is that the bigger your dreams, the bigger your audience of naysayers. Here are the actions that can help you overcome their words of uncertainty.

TRUST YOUR INNER COMPASS.

Why the heck are you going after your goals anyway if there are naysayers saying it's impossible? I don't know about you, but every time I have pursued something more for myself, it has been because of an inner knowing that this was the right path. I can feel it the moment I start to visualize what life might look like on the other side of the dream. There's a space in my midsection where I can feel my energy light up when I take action in the direction I am meant to move. I must trust that feeling if I am going to actively combat naysayers.

I truly believe that every person has this sense of inner knowing. However, many people will believe they don't because they've ignored it for so long. They've ignored it in favor of the unsupportive partner or in-law. They've ignored it in favor of societal expectations. They've ignored it because they're afraid going boldly toward their dreams would make other people in their lives uncomfortable with their indecision or inaction. Or they've ignored it because they're too tuned out doomscrolling to notice.

Your inner compass is a key source of confidence. While trying something new or going after a big dream may be scary, challenging, or frustrating, when I can tap into my deepest sense that this path is the right path, I can find the confidence to overcome whatever life or naysayers throw my way.

If you have big plans but also naysayers around you, it's time to get in contact with your inner compass. The best way I know to locate your inner compass is to find time and space to do things that bring you unattached joy, meaning activities that you find joyful regardless of what anyone else thinks. Whether that's digging in your garden, skiing down a hill, running at sunrise, or sitting and reading a good book, these moments of true joy are like the magic key that opens up your heart to sense what you really feel is true.

Pay attention to what this unattached joy feels like. Does it feel like a calm across your body? Does it feel like the softness of a warm and cozy blanket? Does it feel like a massive grin on your face? Does it feel like freedom? When you get to know this feeling, you can start to tap into the sensations that show up in your body when you're on the right path in your life. Your body will draw you toward the actions that are in alignment with yourself. When you continually tap into that wisdom, it doesn't mean you will no longer feel like your mouth is full of cotton balls during public speaking. Nor will it make fundraising for an important cause feel less like an uphill slog.

What listening to your inner knowing does is enable enough trust in yourself that you're willing to continue to act despite the resistance of naysayers. The most important thing that I have found to combat naysayers' glances and words is action. The most important thing I have found to keep me working even when it's hard, boring, or downright scary is to connect back to the feeling in my body that vibrates when I am on the right track. That feeling will remind me on a day that I don't want to take action that one small step is still a step in the right direction and one that proves the naysayers wrong.

FALL IN LOVE WITH THE PROCESS.

There is a common human trait that makes us think we need to delay our gratification and joy until the moment we accomplish something. If you're pursuing something that is going to take months or years, that is a long time to persevere for a short moment of gratification. If you're delaying gratification until the end, it's also much easier to want to give up and give in to the naysayers' narrative that you can't accomplish the goal. The antidote to long-suffering is to instead find your joy in the *process* of accomplishing your goals, not the outcome.

In my journey, I found each completion of a semester of coursework or passing a big exam to be very motivating. Writing papers was hard work, but it felt empowering to see the completed product. The day-to-day work of grinding through studying was exhilarating because I knew I was making progress toward the bigger goal, my PhD. Further, I loved who I was becoming in the process. Each day that I showed up to do the work, I became more resilient and a better wife, mom, and colleague. If I would have attached my joy to the outcome of a PhD in hand, I would have missed out on all the joy and growth that occurred during the process.

When you tie your expectations to the outcome alone, it is very easy to get frustrated by how long it is taking. Instead, try attaching your expectations to how much time you need to put in every day or small milestones. This way, you get to celebrate your success regularly rather than deciding to be happy when it is all over. Falling in love with the process means falling into bed feeling accomplished rather than defeated or with dread at another day of hard work ahead.

What's your big goal? What is your equivalent to pursuing a PhD? The thing that popped into your head when you read that sentence is your ultimate outcome. To find joy in the process, you must stay present in the process. To stay present in the process, you need a road map of mini-milestones and daily steps toward where you're going.

If your goal is a multiyear project, first you need to know your increment of accomplishment. For example, a PhD is a multiyear process, but we had semesters and exam milestones to mark our incremental movement forward. Second, you need to break down the work within the smaller segment into something your brain can fully hold on to—like a week. Within that week, how much time do you need to invest in your goal? Or within that week, what small milestone, like an exam, do you need to complete? Finally, break that week down day by day. The calendar planning tool mentioned in the previous chapter can be a helpful, concrete way to do this.

I have one *critical* piece of advice to keep yourself motivated on this long trek toward your big goal. Your day-to-day list must be feasible to accomplish in the time you have available to you that day (barring an unknown emergency). If you consistently do not accomplish what you set out to do that day, you will strip the joy and satisfaction from your process. This happens because our brain focuses on what we didn't do regardless of the number of things we did do. For example, if you know you have thirty minutes to dedicate to your goal one day, then the task(s) allotted for that day must be doable in thirty minutes. Save the things that take more time for another day.

If you find yourself slipping into frustration or apathy because things aren't moving as quickly as you'd like or you've become more invested in the outcome than the process, find your way back to that inner compass. Step away mentally and physically long enough to reconnect with that feeling of joy. Then, from that space, reconnect with working the process toward your big goal.

I am not going to sugarcoat it. Big goals take a lot of work and a lot of hours. Most days, you'll feel like you're grinding it out. Working toward a big goal can also get very monotonous. It can seem as slow as molasses. But if you throw the big goal out there, set a plan, work your plan, and wholeheartedly love living that plan, you're going to get to the finish line. You will also learn to love who you are becoming in the process. You're going to accomplish something others thought was impossible.

REFLECTION PROMPTS:

- Who has implicitly or explicitly stated their opposition to your goals? What do you think are the reasons behind their naysaying?
- What makes you want to continue pursuing your goals despite others' opinions?
- What does total joy feel like in your body? How might you tap into that feeling to get to know your inner compass better?
- How have you been delaying your own joy by focusing on outcomes? What might you gain from loving the process?
- What are the next few milestones toward your bigger goal? How might you break these down into weekly and daily tasks?

RESOURCES:

Calendar planning template available at **www.kaseyboehmer.com.**

"Your inner compass is a key source of confidence."

ANTIDOTES FOR

Burnout

In 2019, the eleventh revision of the International Classification of Diseases included burnout as an *occupational phenomenon.*[1] It's important to note that despite this inclusion, it is not considered a medical condition. In short, this classification defines burnout as chronic occupational stress that has not been successfully managed and includes three dimensions: emotional exhaustion, feelings of being disconnected from yourself and your identity, and reduced personal accomplishment.[2]

Less than a year after this designation, our entire world would be turned upside down due to COVID-19. Burnout suddenly became top of mind for everyone, from healthcare workers to educators and remote-learning students, to suddenly work-from-home employees, to parents that now added "homeschool instructor" to their résumés. Yet, let's be honest, many people were suffering from symptoms of burnout pre-pandemic. The pandemic just turned them into a tidal wave, and I would venture to guess that many people still have not recovered from the excessive burnout and trauma caused by the pandemic. We took an already fast-paced world, with a "do more, rest less" attitude, and poured on top of it the trauma of the most significant public health crisis in a century. As we discuss burnout, I also want you to know that I choose to be liberal in my definition of "occupational" as it pertains to the definition of burnout. While many think of occupation as related to one's job(s) or paid work, definitions of one's occupation include "an activity in which one engages" or "the principal business of one's life." As such, your occupations could include studying, caregiving, volunteering, or homemaking, instead of or including paid employment. I think this inclusive definition is important as you reflect on whether you are currently experiencing burnout or have experienced burnout in your past. No one is immune to burnout. I confess, I truly love my work to the extent that the lines between work and homelife can get fuzzy. Prior to my IC/BPS diagnosis, I would stay up past when my kids and husband went to bed to finish reading one more thing related to my work. Now I know better. I know that my body cannot handle that. However, I still am often contemplating my work outside of working hours. Just the other day, I missed my exit while driving because I was internally working on my to-do list.

It is easier to think that if we love our occupation we won't burn out. There is a pervasive saying in our culture that "if you love your work, you'll never work a day in your life." I fundamentally disagree, because as dreamers, movers, shakers, hustlers of the world, we want to do it all. We thrive on doing as much as we can, as best we can, and as hard as we can. We translate many inputs into incredible outputs. And when people see those outputs on our résumés or social media feed, they certainly don't think we could burn out. The problem is that as the goal-getters of the world, we keep taking on new inputs, despite never letting go of others, and suddenly we're completely overcommitted. Once we're overcommitted, it's extremely easy to forget to be mindful and present within our lives so that we can derive joy from the work we're doing. This lack of presence and connection to our work is a recipe for burnout.

For me, the nag of burnout creeping into my soul feels like my energy is being pulled in a million directions and I can't possibly drop one thing. Yet, I also feel like one wrong move, and I will drop it all. Ultimately, this tugging of energy depletes the mind, the spirit, and, eventually, the body. I call this the burnout trifecta.

Have you felt this too? Can you think of a time when the occupational exhaustion started to set in and deposit cobwebs of negativity into your brain? Suddenly, mentally and spiritually you felt like a shell of your former self with no way out. Physically, the manifestations of burnout are different for everyone. For me, burnout and exhaustion are bad news for the chronic conditions I live with, because as I mentioned before, stress can trigger symptom flare-ups. You may or may not have that challenge. Nevertheless, there is a strong connection between our minds and bodies. Meaning, even if you don't have a formal medical condition, burnout can still bring about physical manifestations such as headaches, digestion issues, poor sleep, or a general sense of feeling unwell.

What do we do when we hit burnout status? Well, at the beginning of adulthood, I'd just push through any mental, physical, or emotional symptoms of burnout. No matter what fire was burning or building was collapsing, I would go through heroic efforts to keep getting through all the things I was trying to juggle. As I have grown in my life and career, I have realized that this is not an option that is sustainable. I cannot simply power through the heavy blanket of what burnout feels like. I need my mind to be free to problem-solve; burnout stifles that. I need my spirit to be free to dream big dreams; burnout stifles that too. And if I am not careful to stop it in its tracks, the stress of burnout will cause my body to revolt. Physical pain and bone-deep fatigue are the ultimate result of not letting myself rest.

Here's a good rule of thumb when you're thinking about your own propensity toward burnout: when you feel like you should push the gas pedal to try to keep up with all the deadlines, asks, and work, that is exactly when you need to pump the brakes. Here are some ways that I have found are particularly useful in pumping the brakes and pulling myself out of a phase of burnout.

A STAYCATION.

Sometimes when you're burned out, planning a vacation that requires you to go somewhere might actually feel overwhelming. Yet, a vacation can be a highly effective component of a burnout intervention. My solution to this challenge has been to do staycations instead of going-somewhere vacations.

Staycations are fantastic for a number of reasons when you're burnt out. You don't have to activate your brain to pack a suitcase with everything you need or deal with the stress of airports or long car trips. There is no need to dress up, and you can even stay in your pajamas and fuzzy robe all day if you really want to. Staycations don't cost a thing if you don't want them to, but if you want to splurge a little, you can take yourself out to lunch or engage in some activity of self-care like getting a massage. You might want to do the things on your life to-do list that have been stagnating because your work to-do list has been too long or overwhelming. These activities might include tidying up your space, doing laundry, or attending doctor appointments. But mostly, if you really want to, you can do *absolutely nothing* for a few days or, *gasp*, a whole week!

Staycations are my number-one line of defense against burning out from all the things I pursue at one time. I typically build them into my schedule, so that I get at least one in the summer and one in the winter. When I take them, I shut off work like it doesn't even exist. I don't even check email. Yes, I have about five hundred messages waiting for me when I get back, but I feel rested to take them on, and in some cases, I don't need to do anything because another coworker took care of the matter while I was out.

And just a reminder, I love my work! I love it all, and it fills my soul with the knowledge that I am doing what I was uniquely put on the earth to do. You know what, though? No matter how much I love it, I still need a break from it. So, when you begin to feel that you're burning out, even in the midst of doing something you love, stop feeling guilty for putting everything down for a minute to focus on you and your recovery. Do not ever doubt the power of your couch, fuzzy socks, and a good nap in the battle against burnout.

REMIND YOURSELF WHY YOU STARTED.

For me, usually after a break and a week away from the grind, I begin to feel the tug of my heartstrings back toward my calling. Rather than feeling emotionally exhausted or negative about the work that lies ahead of me, I begin to want it again. There are several reasons for me: I can feel the ways in which my research is helping other people with chronic conditions. I also feel deeply motivated as a woman and a mother working in science to demonstrate that possibility to up-and-coming female scientists. I also enjoy the progress of seeing a paper published, a grant funded, one of my students successfully graduating, or a patient I'm coaching make their own breakthrough. There are many aspects to my work that I feel a deep attachment to but that I can begin to feel detachment to when I'm experiencing burnout.

For you, your job, your studies, and/or your side hustle is yours for a reason. Whatever it is, you have a reason you started *this thing*. Not another thing. Not the thing you think you want to do next. Now it's time to go back and reflect on that starting line again. You may have started this occupation because of the passion you had for it. But that may not be the case. Sometimes you start something because it's the only way you can see yourself getting out of a negative situation—maybe your occupation gave you the opportunity to escape an unhealthy relationship and financially sustain yourself on your own. Whatever the reason you began, connecting back to that starting point can refresh your outlook to help you recover from burnout so you can continue or complete the tasks.

In the hustle and bustle of everyday life, it is easy to lose sight of that original drive. This is especially true if what you're pursuing is a long haul to the finish line, or something that doesn't have a clear finish line. Pursuing a degree or certification takes a long time. Paying off debt, becoming financially independent, or starting a family are all long-term endeavors. Pursuing greatness in your life never stops. In the long game, motivation and positivity can wane, which can contribute to burnout in a major way.

Take a moment to think back to the very beginnings of the endeavor that is making you feel burned out now and try to remember how you felt then. Did you feel excitement? Maybe some butterflies in your stomach? Did you feel inspired? Did you feel good about starting down this path? Did it feel hard but necessary? Once you've connected with those original feelings, sit with them for a bit and think about where there may have been a disconnect between that starting point and where you are now. Taking a moment to let your soul simmer in that feeling of what it was like in the beginning can spark memories and emotions that are a strong antidote for the symptoms of burnout. If it comes to a point you cannot reconnect with any good aspect of what you're doing, then maybe it is time to say goodbye to it for good. And if that's the case, make sure the next thing you start has a solid reason behind it.

IDENTIFY WHAT YOUR SITUATION IS TRYING TO TEACH YOU.

Finally, we know that building muscle in our bodies requires workouts and proper nutrients. Often, getting these workouts and nutrients in our life doesn't feel particularly enjoyable. Similarly, building a phenomenal life requires some soul workouts and proper self-growth nutrients, particularly if we want to bounce back from feeling disconnected or unaccomplished in our occupation. The hardships you're going through right now might just be your soul workout that builds your stamina for the next challenge. The challenges you're facing in this moment that have you wanting to quit might just be pulling you toward what you need to do to take your life to the next level.

When I'm going through a difficult situation, my favorite question to ask myself is, "How is this happening for me, not to me?" If this challenge is happening to me, I am getting battered and beat down by it. But if instead it is happening for me, I am gaining something from the process even if the process isn't particularly enjoyable.

I have experienced this kind of soul workout in the past. In 2018, after I completed my PhD, I applied for a promotion to faculty at my institution. This promotion required I demonstrate full grant funding for at least three years, a lengthy packet of papers (including my résumé and letters of recommendation), and a forty-five-minute oral presentation of my research. This process took about a year to complete. When it came time to talk to the division chair about my position, I was informed that the committee had decided I was not yet ready to move to the faculty ranks. I was absolutely devastated. I felt like a complete wreck, and yet I had to hold it somewhat together to walk back to my office full of my colleagues eager to hear the outcome of my meeting.

After I broke the news, I went to the gym and ran on the treadmill. I cried most of that run, from anger, despair, and disappointment. I was angry that I had gone through a year of the process only to be told no. I was in despair because it felt like everything I had worked for over the span of nine years was slipping away. I was disappointed in that I'd never had something so big fall through. I went home to my family and cried some more. Truly, I mean it when I say that was the worst day of my professional career. It's very difficult to not feel burnt out after a grueling process and public failure.

After the shock finally dissipated, I had to seriously consider what to do next. Did I want to try this again at my institution, knowing I could again be told I wasn't ready? Or did I want to quit trying there and apply for positions elsewhere? I realized I could also be turned down somewhere else, but I knew it wouldn't hurt as much as the previous process had. While some folks might wonder if I ever thought of quitting research, I didn't. I hadn't labored for ten years pursuing a PhD to walk away from the career that meant so much to me.

Ultimately, what did I decide to do? I asked myself the question of all questions. "How is this happening for me, not to me?" I determined that I knew the process, so I could be better prepared the second time around. I knew the people who were part of the selection process, so I could meet with them to ask them what I needed to work on. I would ultimately be a better mentor having gone through this process. I had colleagues who stood by me and guided me, even at my lowest. In the end, I put my head down, did the work for another year, and tried again. The second time around, I was successful, to the point the same committee told me I'd knocked it out of the park.

That second year of work, meetings, repetition, and focus was tough, especially coming off a mentally grueling letdown. Ultimately, though, I persevered, and so I know you can too. To do so, I need you to shift your focus. I need you to write down five reasons that what you are doing right now is happening for you. I am quite sure that you, like me during that hard letdown, have rehearsed a hundred times how this situation has happened to you. But have you ever thought about the fact that your next position, your next relationship, your next phase in life might not be here yet because you haven't learned what you need to learn in this hard phase, right here, right now? Think about how much work a seed needs to do to sprout, how much work an animal needs to do to survive winter, or how much a rock needs to endure to become a diamond. How is this moment shaping the next version of you? I'm cheering you on—you got this.

REFLECTION PROMPTS:

- How does burnout show up for you mentally, spiritually, and physically?
- What are your body's cues to let you know you're headed for exhaustion, negativity, or reduced abilities?
- What would carving out time in the near future for rest look like to you? How about carving out time way in advance for rest and recovery?
- What are the reasons you started the endeavor for which you are now losing steam? Do those motivations still resonate with you?
- How might the challenges you're facing right now be for you? What are they teaching you?

"When you feel like you should push the gas pedal to try to keep up with all the deadlines, asks, and work, that is exactly when you need to pump the brakes."

ANTIDOTES FOR

Complacency

It was the fall of 2017. My health was finally stable, a year and a half into my IC/BPS diagnosis. I was beginning my dissertation year, which might sound hard, but in reality, the coursework that ate my nights and weekends was over. For me, fitting all the classes into my busy schedule was the hardest part of the PhD process. My dissertation aligned with the work I was already doing, and so the writing felt relatively easy. Ultimately, I thought I had everything figured out for my next steps.

What I did not have figured out and couldn't see from within my circumstances was that the fall and winter of 2017 and the spring of 2018 were seasons of plateau for me. Plateauing on the roller coaster of life is equivalent to coasting. Hitting a plateau means you are no longer being challenged. And remember, you need challenges to grow. You need adversity to shape you. In other words, plateaus lead to complacency, which, if we allow it to continue for too long, is a problem if we hope to become something better than what we are today.

Complacency is a challenge for even the biggest achievers, but it's worth distinguishing first from burnout. Complacency feels comfortable, like you've finally settled into the blankets on your couch on a cold winter day and it's so comfortable you never want to get up. It's a sense of quiet contentment. You have no reason to purposefully pull yourself from it when you reach it. Burnout, on the other hand, feels like you're running on a hamster wheel as fast as you can but still not keeping up. You feel exhausted and cynical about what lies in front of you because you have no gas or love left in the tank. Burnout feels like something you very much would like to escape by pulling the blankets over your head and hiding for days, yet you can't because you feel the need to keep running. We're talking about the former cozy comfort here, not complete exhaustion.

You will likely confront complacency at least once, if not more, in early adulthood. This happens because at some point in very early adulthood, you set off on more independent adventures like work, college, or both. This typically requires you to calibrate to new schedules, new responsibilities, new goals, and new activities. There may be additional periods of major adjustment should you also decide to begin a committed partnership or start a family. All these changes that occur in a relatively short span of time really push you past your comfort zone and make you figure things out on your feet. These challenges make it hard to be in a place of complacency. However, once you adjust to them, you're likely to hit points where you start to coast. Should you want to continue a trajectory of growth as you move forward in adulthood, when embedded challenges become less frequent, you will need to be more intentional about your plans for growth. In other words, that couch feels very warm and cozy, but you're not going to expand your horizons from there.

The following questions can also help you sort out if you have plateaued in your growth.

1. Does everything feel easy? How long has it felt that way? I mean truly easy—not that you are in a state of flow, where things are challenging but getting done rapidly.
2. Do you have any activities that are new or fresh in some way on your calendar? These could be work activities, social activities, family activities, personal hobbies, etc.
3. Do you have any items on your to-do list that challenge you? I am not necessarily talking about the kind of challenge that requires you to mentally overcome not wanting to do a given task. I am talking about the kind of challenge that you know will take some time and mental effort to make happen.
4. How many days a week are you doing at least one thing outside your usual comfort zone? These things could be big, such as giving a new presentation to a large audience, or small, such as saying hello to one new person in a social setting.

Now look at your list. If you answered *yes* to number 1, *no* to numbers 2 and 3, and *not very often* or *never* to number 4, that means you are meeting my primary diagnostic criteria for a plateau. In this case, it is probably worth considering if you're plateauing or not. Are you challenging yourself in all the ways you want to be challenging yourself? Upon learning this, some people may feel immediately uncomfortable, because high achievers typically never want to be in a plateau; others may think, "What's so bad about life feeling easy?"

There is nothing inherently wrong with easy—but it won't challenge or change you for the better. Think of a sprouting plant again, stretching its sweet little limbs toward the sky and the light. Nothing about its growth has been easy, from the cracking open of its seed to it finally emerging above the soil. If it wants to continue to grow, it must reach toward the sunlight with all its might, because there are other plants that want to crowd it out to get more light too. If the plant no longer reaches for more light, its growth will be stunted, and the other plants will overcrowd it to its detriment. Imagine yourself as the plant, choosing to become complacent about the light to which you're exposed. You're going to plateau in the form of not growing, being overshadowed, or being crowded out. This means a freezing in place in terms of your joy, your impact, your success, your income, and so on. If you don't want to be stuck where you are, you're going to have to get out of this plateau.

Is it never OK to be in a plateau? Not necessarily. If your plateau comes after a season of serious growth or burnout, a short reprieve can give you space to catch your breath for a minute and rest. However, as soon as you start to feel frustrated that you're not experiencing growth mentally, physically, emotionally, or spiritually, it's time to get back in action. In my experience, the end of a plateau is typically signaled by my thinking, "OK, what's next?" Your ability to coax yourself out of a comfortable plateau and back into growing might be assisted by the following ideas.

REMEMBER, YOU ARE LIMITLESS.

My mom always told me: "Never tell a child what their limits are;

let them show you." What she meant was that parents, teachers, coaches, and society are often giving children messages about their capabilities. For example, if a child is a first grader, there are certain things that first graders are supposed to do, and of course, if they struggle to do them, they may need extra time, attention, and resources to ensure they continue to develop. However, people often put boundaries around what first grade kids can and should do.

If you tell a first grader that he can only read first grade books, he will only read first grade books. If you tell a sixth grader that certain math problems are for her junior high years, she will save those problems for her junior high years. If you tell a child that certain sports skills will be developed when he or she is eleven, they will wait to try those skills until they are eleven. Or, if they try them early and fall short, they will stop striving for them, since logically, they will surmise that those skills are reserved for age eleven.

It's no different for adults. If you tell yourself that you cannot do something because you didn't meet a prerequisite, you will either not try at all or try it once; if you fail, you will decide that the failure wasn't because it was your first try but because you didn't meet the prerequisite. And then you'll quit trying. A good example of this is when you see a job opening for the next level within your career and it lists a suggested number of years of experience. When you see that suggested number of years and you haven't met it, do you go ahead and apply or not even bother?

What if, instead, you approach a job or a skill that is new and hard as an opportunity available to anyone and everyone? With this mindset, sure, you may fail, but you won't assume it is because of your limited abilities. Instead, you will try again. *Let me be very clear—your goals and dreams don't have limits.* When everyone else, including you, seems to think that there are limits, you need to remind yourself—you are limitless.

How does this idea apply to your plateau? Well, sometimes life is going to force you out of complacency. It's going to force you into a hard place of heartbreak, grief, illness, or struggle. However, in other cases, you're going to want to find growth without being forced to. Sometimes, you're going to want to choose to level up.

Leveling up when your hand is not forced is possible only if you're in the right mindset. If your mindset has imposed limits to your potential, breaking out of your plateau requires knocking down those limits. Your potential is limitless, as long as you believe that is true. Stop telling yourself the equivalent of first graders can only read first grade books. Life is for everyone. Tell me what you're ready for in your life. I guarantee that you just had a pretty wild dream pop into your head, but you may have silenced it immediately with something along the lines of, "No, I'm not ready for that," or, "There are so many steps I have to take first before I get there."

So freaking what?! Yes, I am fired up about this! Every single person that does incredible things in this world was once a beginner. They once said, "I want to try that," and then they did. They once were clunky singers, athletes, financiers, and students. Yet some of those people decided to stick it out and keep practicing their craft. They often failed; their audition wasn't successful, they didn't make the team, or their business decision flopped. However, they didn't stop practicing and pursuing their goals. People who don't try things often assume they will be terrible at it; they assume every talented person they see started with the proficiency they observe now. This is called a fixed mindset.[1] The thought that you will be terrible at first is likely true, but the only path from failure to success is to try to practice diligently. This is called a growth mindset.[1] The time will pass anyway; why not pass it working toward what you really want? Stop limiting your potential. Stop hanging out in the plateau.

UP YOUR PERSONAL DEVELOPMENT GAME.

Focusing on personal development is the secret sauce in getting the most out of life and breaking through your plateaus. Meaningful personal development activities can help you tap into that inner compass and are what you should be focusing on next. For me, the most meaningful personal development practices in my life are journaling, spending time with a biblical devotional, and prayer. As a spiritual person, these activities help me access my intuition and decide what I want next in my life. It is important that you experiment with what could be meaningful practices in your life too, and they don't have to be spiritual if that isn't your belief system.

Given that all of us have different comfort zones and we're each currently in different seasons of life, you will have your own preferred medium when it comes to personal development. Here are some ideas for more personal development activities: vision casting; reading nonfiction books, listening to podcasts, or taking courses (academic/nonacademic); meditating or practicing mindfulness; engaging in coaching, counseling, or therapy; learning a new skill or hobby; or resurrecting an old hobby that you haven't taken time to do in a long while.

If you don't have any that come to mind yet, don't try everything at once. The idea isn't to overwhelm yourself, but rather to develop a toolbox of things over a period of time that can help you grow when you feel stuck. It is totally fine to pick one activity and focus on it or do multiple different activities at a time. Whatever floats your boat. If you can, I would suggest committing sixty minutes each day (and they don't have to be consecutive minutes) to personal development. However, if this is completely new for you, I would encourage you to start by finding one thing to focus on and ten minutes a day to do it. Then you can build from that foundation. Those ten minutes could be early in the morning before everyone else wakes up, during your commute to work or school, or before you go to bed. Pick whatever works for you and commit to it. Commit to the first ten minutes, and when that begins to feel like a habit and you're wanting more, add more time.

If I had to recommend a starting place, it would be vision casting, as I think this is a great foundational activity. Vision casting is the act of intentionally considering where you want to be and what you want to feel like in life at some future point in time. Some people will do this in meditation, others on a vision board, and others in written form in a journal.

When was the last time you thought about what you want in the next week, days, months, years? You kind of need to know where you're going, because stringing days together without a vision is going to get you somewhere that does not feel like your wildest dreams. (Not that detours are always bad, but if you continually end up somewhere on the map so far from where you wanted to be, you're going to get frustrated.) If you have an idea of where you're going, you have a much better chance of getting there.

I can already hear what you may be thinking. "Oh my gosh, I am barely scraping by," or "I can't pay all my bills," or "I don't even have a car," or whatever your current situation may be. You may feel like you need to focus on that before you can indulge in this vision casting thing I'm talking about. So, let me say this with a whole lot of love: vision casting *is. not. a. luxury.*

Your vision can be living a life where you pay your bills on time and have a steady mode of transportation. There is no judgment for your dreams. Because if that's what you know you want and need in your life, and you go all in, I'm here to cheer you on. Your vision, no matter what it looks like, is inviting you to leave your complacency and step into something bigger.

Once you know what your vision is and you're ready to take action toward it, you're going to need to pick what activities are going to move you closer to what you want in life. In doing this, you need to encircle yourself with positive, growth-minded people and creative problem solvers. If you have those kinds of people in your life, certainly you're a step ahead of the game. However, if you don't have those kinds of influences, that is OK too, because you can find positive, growth-minded teachers in books, podcasts, social media, courses, conferences, etc.

Those are the "who" that will help you reach up and out of your plateau. To determine the "what" that will help you move forward, you need to ask yourself, "What activity or activities would I need to do regularly to move in the direction of the vision for my future self?" Maybe you want to read up on a skill you want to learn, enroll in a new course, or map out your ideas on paper.

The great news is that basically anything you want in life is teachable. You want more confidence? Teachable. You want to learn how to ice skate? Teachable. You need more grounding spiritually? Teachable. You want to learn how to do finances because you're twenty years into adulthood and still struggle with them? No problem, also teachable. Whatever it is you want in your life, there is a resource out there somewhere, often free or at minimal cost, to at least dip your toes into what will help you get there. You *just* need to carve out the time and commitment to finding it and acting upon it.

I say *just* because anyone who has tried anything new in the midst of a busy life knows that simply carving out time, commitment, and action isn't quite as simple as it sounds. It's easy to come up with excuses for why engaging in personal development won't fit into your already busy life or isn't for you. You may get hung up on what others might think about you changing your routines and trying something new. You might get tripped up in thinking that an expanded life isn't for you because it feels like nothing has gone in your favor. You might simply say no to expanding your life in personal development because it feels scary or impossible for where you're at. The first step always feels the hardest. Our brains are wired to keep us safe and comfortable for our survival. Therefore, our brains often favor going with the crowd, staying in a familiar location, and doing things that don't extend our energy beyond our current capacity. Seeking discomfort through personal development is taking an active step against what our brain feels like it should be doing. That's always going to be hard. Try the ten minutes a day for three days as an experiment. If you don't like the activity, you can switch to another one or quit altogether, but that thirty minutes total might give you a new perspective that you'll want to explore further.

Much of what I've talked about here is for someone who is fairly new to the idea of personal development. Some folks might be longtime personal developers in a plateau. If that is you, I want you to shake things up a little. For example, if you've been reading a particular author or attending a particular class a lot, it's probably time to try a new one or even switch up your medium. For example, switch from a book to a podcast. Personal development is a lifelong engagement, so if you're already a seasoned veteran at it and you're in a plateau, you're going to need to be more intentional about this activity. It is not possible to take in the same personal development content repeatedly and expect to continue growing. Pushing your boundaries and getting uncomfortable isn't a bad thing—it's just not something we always like. Buckle up and bust out of your comfort zone to find that next level you're seeking.

REFLECTION PROMPTS:

- Based on the diagnostic criteria above, are you currently in a plateau? If so, how long have you been in this place?
- If you're in a plateau, are you happy being here to rest and recover, or are you anxious for what is next?
- What limits have you placed on yourself that may be keeping you in your comfort zone? Where do those limiting beliefs come from?
- What is one action that you could take now that is in opposition to your limiting beliefs? What is one small step you can take that moves you out of your plateau space?
- What, if any, personal development activities are you currently doing? What activities might you want to explore to up your personal development game?

"The time will pass anyway; why not pass it working toward what you really want?"

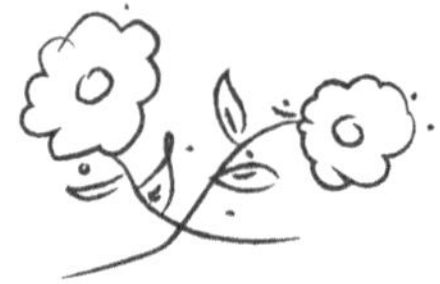

PART III

ANTIDOTES FOR

Juggling Work and Family

On April 9, 2011, I married the love of my life, Jeff Boehmer. In 2012, we welcomed our first child, Owen. In 2020, as ever-stronger partners and seasoned parents of an eight-year-old, we welcomed our second child, Oscar. I grew up with two married, loving parents who very much have been part of our nuclear family since Owen's birth. My dad remains in that role, but my mother passed away from cancer in 2018, leaving a big hole in all our hearts. She taught me how to be a mama, and I try to remember those lessons every day. I have done many awesome things in my life, but this sweet, loving family will always be by far my greatest accomplishment.

Based on this description, you can tell I have what might be described as a "traditional" family by a previous generation's standards. Nowadays, I think families look much more diverse, and I think that is for the better. It's worth noting the perspective I take, because the challenges I discuss are layered with the privilege of a heterosexual nuclear family. If you are coming from a nontraditional family that doesn't have some of these majority privileges, the challenges of balancing work and family may have additional layers of struggle, or you may have new ones altogether. No matter what it looks like, there is likely a time in early adulthood where you'll establish a family of some sort. This family may include any combo of partner, pets, kids, biological family, married-into family, chosen family, and/or friends. To me, the defining features of a family are: 1) you care deeply enough about these people that you would regularly choose to put their needs ahead of your own; 2) you have some responsibility of care for them; and 3) you spend, through in-person or digital interaction, significant amounts of time with them regularly.

Where I am today and where I was ten years ago when I first established a family are vastly different. These days people often look at me as a woman who "does it all." Years ago, I became a mother at the ripe old age of twenty-two. I was still establishing my own identity and learning how to be a good partner. I can readily admit, I had absolutely no idea what I was doing, even if I wanted to do it all.

Let me tell you, if you haven't experienced it, bringing a newborn into your life will rock your world. Suddenly, this very teeny tiny being needs you every second of every day just to stay alive. They eat about every ninety minutes, sleep constantly but also don't know how to sleep without soothing (why?!), and produce more laundry than two grown adults ever could. Quite suddenly, your every waking and sleeping need is downgraded in importance to your newborn's every waking and sleeping need. And factor in that you are tired to your bones.

I think a good illustration—even if a bit personal—of how my world changed in the months following the birth of Owen was in my experience of choosing to feed him exclusively breast milk. Breastfeeding is a biological means to feed our babies. Thankfully, we have the option of formula or pumping expressed milk now for those who choose not to or who cannot breastfeed exclusively. These modern inventions allow us as women to pursue things outside of tending to our newborns. Without formula or pumping, it would be extremely difficult for women to hold positions in the workplace during their childbearing years. However, given the large proportion of women in the workplace that do have children, I think it is important for us to talk about the experience of needing to organize your entire life around providing nutrition to your baby.

For those unfamiliar from firsthand experience, when you're breastfeeding or pumping, if it works as it is supposed to, you will continue producing milk for your child even if you're not with them. So, while you're doing your working mom thing, you're still constantly producing milk, and if you do not remove said milk, there will be physical pain. Therefore, you organize your entire day around your boobs not screaming at you. You may laugh, but it's true.

Some women pump at work and seamlessly transition to nursing their child when they get home. Unfortunately, that never worked for me, although I tried mightily to force it. The first couple of months of returning to work after Owen's birth were a nightmare of trying to get the timing right so that my boobs weren't screaming at me and the baby wasn't screaming at the caretaker. Eventually, I switched to exclusively pumping. Some people hate "EPing," as it's called, but for me it improved my quality of life significantly.

Until Owen was one years old, I pumped every four or five waking hours. This meant I had to organize my meetings, my workouts, my hangouts, and my graduate school studying around my pumping schedule. The pinnacle of this experience was when Owen was ten months and I left him home with my husband and parents to care for him while I went to a work conference in Peru. By the time I did this, I had found a way to have a structured pumping schedule in my daily life. However, that all went out the window once I was completely taken out of my routine. Suddenly I was in a country where pumping was not the norm and I had no access to pumping spaces outside of my hotel room. I was also on a conference schedule that was nonstop, and I had not considered when I would need to take breaks. At the end of the trip, we visited Machu Picchu, which is an all-day excursion with tourists everywhere, no breaks, and no places to pump. I was so uncomfortable but finally had to sit myself on the bathroom floor by the hand dryer because that was the only semiprivate space I could find. It was really eye-opening trying to juggle these responsibilities—my professional career, my physical needs, and my caretaking tasks—at a distance.

Breastfeeding or pumping is an extreme example of the requirements a working mother may have to fulfill to meet the needs of her family. You will have your own examples of needs that your family has of you. It is not uncommon for me to hear working mothers say they feel guilty when they're home because they're thinking about work, and they feel guilty at work because they're thinking about home. That doesn't feel like a very happy place to be all the time—never feeling like you are doing anything well.

I certainly fell prey to this catch-22 early in motherhood,

but I have found a natural balance for the most part these days. While certainly some of that has come through successful strategies of calendaring and prioritizing, a great deal of it has also come through good communication and working together with my family to balance caregiving and career roles. In many ways this was possible because of my incredibly supportive husband and understanding parents. Among us, we communicate regularly about who is picking up what kid and when someone is planning a trip. We have a nice balance of household chores too. My husband does a great job keeping our home organized on the outside with mowing, snow-blowing, and various repairs. I focus my efforts on the indoor chores like dishes and laundry. My dad is now retired but juggles a lot of caregiving roles, including of my kiddos. We expect to share the load and don't hesitate to ask each other when one of us needs help with something.

As humans, I think we are made to be in service to others, but you must find some balance between serving others and accomplishing your own dreams. That balance is far easier said than done. In fact, I think the balance of family and career pursuits is probably the hardest balancing act you will ever do. Here are some of the strategies that I have used to help me find the right balance.

COMMIT TO ONE ACT OF SELF-CARE A DAY.

In some ways there is a gendered aspect to this advice. It is far more ingrained in women through their upbringing that they are the caretakers. Historically, they have been displayed as the homemakers of the world, and putting others' needs above their own is subtly instilled in girls throughout their childhood and young adulthood. However, to some extent, regardless of your gender, there is a real tendency early in a relationship or parenting to forget who you are or what you did to care for your own well-being outside of caring for a partner or child. And for a while this may be absolutely fine and necessary. However, it becomes an issue when it shifts from a temporary to permanent state.

A common cliché you may hear people tell you is, "You can't pour from an empty cup." And you may think, "Yeah, right, that's nice, but have you seen the state of my life right now?"

Let me reframe this for you. Instead of the empty cup cliché, think of an almost-empty gas tank. If you run your gas down to empty, what will you give your family, friends, and other people you care about?

Fumes.

Fumes will spill out that are cranky, short, tired, depressed, or anxious. These fumes are generated from your last effort at pushing the pedal with insufficient gas in the tank and will be spewed at the people who deserve your love and patience the most. Do you really want to give that to your people?

Truly, I think our greatest calling, regardless of gender, is to serve and love others. This has roots in my Christian faith, but I think that love and service are universal values that transcend religion. Loving and serving means our communities at large, family, friends, and colleagues. I want to give the best version of myself to the people I love, however aspirational that is. I can only do that if I have some gas in my tank. I can't play with my kids, have a conversation with my husband, or invest in any number of housework tasks with an empty tank. What gives me gas in the tank? Things like seven to nine hours of sleep per night, alone time to read something I enjoy, a good workout, healthy food, and giving myself a mani/pedi.

I don't allow myself to consistently run on fumes because if I do, at minimum, I will not give my best self to my family or the world. In the worst-case scenario, I will completely crash out and be of no use to myself or anyone else.

When I say commit to one act of self-care a day, it isn't about some perfect self-care regimen that takes hours. It's often difficult to find that kind of time, especially when juggling work and family. What I have found is that if I consistently put at least one act of self-care near the top of my daily priorities list, instead of always relegating them to the very bottom, I consistently have gas in the tank. This single self-care task is an act of love to me, which spills over to love of others. Actively choosing to move my body for thirty minutes or cook a meal or slowly sip my morning tea before diving into work is enough to keep some fuel reserves.

When I am in an especially busy season with work deadlines or a challenging one where my health conditions are causing me battle fatigue, the notion of doing just one thing is important. Thinking I am going to cook dinner, exercise, and meditate all in the context of a normal day can feel really overwhelming or exhausting during times when the calendar is already jam-packed or I am not feeling my best. Focusing on one small thing ensures that I get it done and I don't feel guilty if other self-care activities don't happen. More isn't always better. In this case, consistency—no matter how simple—is your focus.

Ultimately, doing one act of self-care a day is you telling yourself you are worthy of love and care. When you invest in yourself, even in small ways each day, you become holistically healthy and full of love. That love gets distributed into the lives of your family members. You not only give them the gift of your love, but also demonstrate what it looks like to love yourself and pass that love on to others.

PLAN AND PRIORITIZE YOUR TO-DO LIST.

The challenge when you're living this work-family juggle is twofold. First, you're managing a lot of different moving parts. You are managing tasks related to your employment or business, household, hobbies, and your own schedule as well as that of others. Second, unexpected things come up. A meeting gets added to your calendar last minute. Your kid forgets their backpack, and now you just added twenty extra minutes to your morning drop-off schedule. Inevitably, there will be days when you have to drop something. It's important that you know ahead of the emergency or inconvenience what can get dropped and in what order.

Some things cannot be dropped without calling in backup, such as picking up the kids at school or preparing for a big presentation at work tomorrow. On the other hand, to-do items that can get dropped today and slated for another day are things like working on a deadline that is a month away or organizing a future sleepover for your child and friends. Selecting what to prioritize is directly correlated with the consequences of not getting it done and what your values are. From a consequences standpoint, if a deadline is a hard deadline in which you will lose something tangible, like income, that gets prioritized over a deadline that won't result in losses of income or opportunities. The latter type of deadlines can be renegotiated. In terms of your values, the higher priorities on your list are those that are in the greatest alignment with them. Ideally, we don't deprioritize something that will make us feel out of alignment with our values.

For example, when Owen was starting elementary school, I had been accepted to participate in a conference in London. While it was an incredible opportunity and one I had put effort into applying for, participating would have caused me to miss Owen's first day of kindergarten. So the choice was to either miss out on a great conference opportunity in London, a location I'd never visited, or miss out on that first day of kindergarten. Ultimately, I chose to decline the invitation to the conference. I reasoned that over my career, I would certainly have more opportunities to travel to London. I would never have the chance to make the first day of kindergarten for my firstborn ever again. I value family and important dates with my family more highly than a work opportunity that isn't mandatory. You might have made a different choice for a different reason, and that's OK. The point isn't to pick what someone else would have chosen but to select the thing that you know aligns with your inner compass.

Putting this advice into action means using your calendar and pillars that were first introduced in chapter 7. Typically, my day-to-day non-negotiables are already slated into my calendar, and then I slot in the other tasks in the to-do list in order of their priority. If my pillars are already slated, then I plan my actual "to-do" list, but I am only planning what can be fit in the available time that is not accounted for by the non-negotiables. If I have two hours in my day not spoken for, then I know I can plan for about two hours' worth of other tasks. This isn't a perfect equation because sometimes what you think will take two hours takes four instead. However, over time as you keep your calendar up to date and regularly plan and prioritize your to-do list, your accuracy in predicting the time required for tasks improves.

To some extent, accuracy in your predictions is important over time because it ultimately affects your confidence. Let me explain. If you repeatedly put more on your to-do list than you can accomplish, your brain begins to generate negative self-talk about the undone items. It likes to say things like "There's never enough time in the day," or "If only you were a little less distracted, you'd figure out how to get it all done," or "Other moms can figure out how to juggle these things—why can't you?"

Your brain essentially sees the evidence on paper of the gap between what you said you'd get done and what you actually did, and then creates an unhelpful narrative. Because of this, practicing predicting the amount you can get done in the time you have holds more importance than the completion of the tasks themselves.

However, it is also important to remember that occasionally getting your to-do list/time allotment wrong doesn't spell doom forever. There are key times when you need to ditch the to-do list and reshuffle everything to another time. These instances include when you or someone you care for is sick, either acutely or experiencing an exacerbation of a chronic illness; when an urgent deadline comes up that is the difference between losing and keeping a client; or when you realize you've overdone it and need rest before you burn out physically or mentally. When this inevitable reshuffling occurs, it is particularly important to monitor your self-talk. In such cases, this reprioritizing is a good thing, because in these moments you're practicing self-compassion and grace.

For me, to-do list reshuffling typically happens because either I personally am in a chronic illness flare-up or my kids or husband are unexpectedly ill. In these moments, because I am a goal-getter, I can easily get frustrated by needing to make time for the unexpected. When I do, my brain likes to say, "I don't have time for this," which is incredibly unhelpful since I *have* to make time, and it generates frustration and impatience with myself or my loved ones. I must proactively cultivate self-talk like "Health and family are the most important priorities right now," and "Everything will get done in time, so let things go for today." You want to generate thoughts that are soothing when you're experiencing what feels like the wheels coming off your game plan.

To summarize, successful juggling looks like this:

1. Have a calendar (digital and/or paper) that has spoken-for time noted: meetings, kids' practices, date nights, etc.
2. Review your calendar daily before you plan your to-do list. Calculate approximately how much time you have available.
3. Write tasks in your to-do list that can be accomplished during that amount of time.
4. List the items on your to-do list in order of most important task to least important task. This way if you don't get to everything, what is left are the less important ones.
5. If anything is left undone on today's to-do list, make sure you identify what day and time it should get moved to in the future.
6. Give yourself grace for things that come up and derail your plan. Get them reprioritized to the next available opportunity.

As you move into a phase of life where you're managing the needs of your family alongside your own career or aspirations, your day-to-day life will be constantly evolving. Try to remember to come back to the very basics of self-care and organization. These can be important pillars to hold tight to when the juggling feels overwhelming.

REFLECTION PROMPTS:

- What does your family look like, and what do they need from you in terms of time, attention, and care?
- Write a list of all the things you consider self-care for your soul. Think about ones you did in the past that you may have stopped doing when you started juggling many things. Keep this list handy to make sure you're doing at least one of these each day.
- What are the non-negotiables in your life? Does your calendar reflect that?
- What are the situations that you anticipate will require you to drop everything and reprioritize your to-dos for later?
- Consider how you talk to yourself about your to-do list and accomplishments. Is your self-talk compassionate or critical? If it is the latter, how might you cultivate compassion instead?

"When you invest in yourself, even in small ways each day, you become holistically healthy and full of love."

ANTIDOTES FOR

Preventing and Dealing with Illness

I'm chronically ill. Not like I-constantly-get-colds-and-infections kind of chronically ill. Rather, I have six medical conditions that will not be cured within my lifetime but must instead be managed daily. You might say, "But you don't look sick," which is something those of us with invisible chronic illnesses hear often. However, the truth is that the only reason I don't look sick is because of all the medications I take and treatments I do.

I've come to terms with the humbling fact that my ability to be alive and not bed-bound is dependent on the small pharmacy of medications in my bathroom cabinet. I currently take twelve prescription medications and five supplements every day. I also manage my conditions with complementary medicines like acupuncture and massage. In addition to my primary care clinician, I have four different specialists involved in my care. Sometimes I see a therapist or a health and wellness coach because they can help me cope and stay centered on my overall well-being in the messiness of all the medical stuff.

Looking back, there are some things I wish I would have known before I encountered new chronic illnesses in my adulthood. First, if you have one chronic condition, the likelihood you will develop additional conditions is high, especially as you age; by the time adults reach sixty-five years of age, 75 percent will have multiple chronic conditions.[1] While I was younger than most at the time of my first few diagnoses, it would have helped me feel a bit more at ease knowing that others go through this too, and I was not a total anomaly. Second, with each new diagnosis it really felt like my whole world got turned upside down. Each time, I felt very scared that I wouldn't be able to have the life I wanted because of my latest diagnosis. What I found out from my lived experience is that while it may take time to find new methods and a rhythm to managing a new condition, eventually you do adapt.

Third, I wish I would have fully understood sooner how my mindset about my diagnoses truly mattered, and not in a toxic positivity "everything is dandy" kind of way. I was able to incorporate living with chronic illness as a meaningful component of my life. In many ways I think of my conditions as superpowers because I get to provide new insights to research and education that I wouldn't otherwise be able to. What my research has shown over the years is that you may not love the ways in which you need to adapt to self-manage a disease at first, but the extent to which you can make peace with it can lead to overall success in continuing things, even small ones, that you enjoy despite illness and treatment.[2] Finally, I wish I knew back then that only the person living in your body can guide you in your day-to-day management of your condition(s). It is within your power to know when to rest, make changes, or reach out for support.

When I was diagnosed with IC/BPS in 2016, it was my first new diagnosis in adulthood but my fourth altogether when added on top of my preexisting asthma, severe and life-threatening allergies, and a heart arrythmia, which were all diagnosed in my childhood. After the IC/BPS diagnosis, it took about a year to return to physically feeling somewhat normal again. I was no longer doubled over in pain, and I no longer needed opioid pain medications. I was on long-term medications to manage the bladder condition. I still, to this day, have "flares," or instances where my symptoms become more noticeable, but by the one-year mark I knew how to manage them. The ability to self-manage was critical, so my symptoms were no longer massively interfering with my day-to-day life.

From a personal chronic care standpoint, 2017 to 2020 was calm for me. Then two important things occurred in 2021 within a couple months of each other. First, I decided to discontinue one of my IC/BPS medications, due to new cautions about its impact on eyesight after continued use.[3] As a result of this decision, I experienced the worst IC/BPS flare since my initial diagnosis. Second, I stopped breastfeeding my second baby, Oscar. Within two months of stopping breastfeeding, I began to experience new symptoms that were autoimmune in nature. Autoimmune conditions are ones in which a person's own body develops antibodies against its own tissue. There is long-standing evidence that these diseases are most experienced by people assigned female at birth, and there are unique risks to developing new or flaring existing autoimmune diseases during the pregnancy and postpartum period.[4] Not all mechanisms for these changes are clear. However, pregnancy initiates important changes to the immune system that keeps it from attacking the baby in the womb. The postpartum period, including breastfeeding, also causes changes in the immune system and its responses.[4]

When I first began experiencing new symptoms, I initially thought it was an acute illness. The week after the Fourth of July holiday in 2021, I came down with what seemed to be the world's worst case of pink eye. My eyes were completely swollen shut in the mornings. They were itchy, sticky, and hot. My sensitivity to light was so bad that I had to wear sunglasses even in the house. My husband and I joked I was in my diva phase.

After antibiotics and a few weeks of recovery, the pink eye seemed to go away. Until a few weeks later, it was back again. And then again. After the third time around, I couldn't ignore the fact that whatever was going on was not a typical acute case of pink eye my baby brought home from day care. Soon, a blanket of fatigue set in, and this was combined with the pain I was already trying to manage from my IC/BPS flare. I was also having breathing difficulty that seemed somewhat different from my normal asthma symptoms. Suddenly, with all this going on in my body, walking up the stairs with a load of laundry felt almost impossible. I would have to take a break each time I did. This was not particularly ideal for a busy, constantly needed mother of a newborn and older child. I felt miserable physically. But I also felt that way emotionally as things I needed and wanted to do became more difficult. There was simply no way to will my body to move forward. I also had some panic that was setting in about how I would be able to deal with the work of seeking a new diagnosis. This was only magnified when I thought of what would happen if I actually got a new diagnosis. I knew how much effort it took to get my life back from my IC/BPS experience. I constantly felt like screaming into the abyss: "What is happening to my body?!"

While I pursued consults with my asthma doctor, my bladder doctor, and a new eye doctor—asking all of them, "Isn't it weird this is all happening at once?"—they seemed to think it was just bad luck and unfortunate timing. I was skeptical. I've had chronic illness flares my whole life, but they never happened so simultaneously and ferociously. On my own intuition, I asked for a consult with a rheumatologist, a doctor that handles autoimmune conditions. My hunch was based on the knowledge from my previous reading when I was diagnosed with IC/BPS that there was a correlation between it and Sjögren's syndrome, an autoimmune disease.[5]

My skepticism was warranted, and after a significant battery of tests, I was diagnosed with Sjögren's syndrome in September 2021. Sjögren's causes the body to mistakenly attack your exocrine glands, or the glands that produce moisture like your tears or saliva. Typically, people have dry eyes, sometimes to the point of chronic pink eye like I experienced, and dry mouth. Additionally, many other patients also have other symptoms like fatigue, lung difficulties, or neuropathy, which is nerve damage that can cause numbness or pain, usually in the extremities. I began treatment with corticosteroids to calm the inflammation and immunosuppressants to calm my immune system's military-grade attack on my own body. Things got better, almost normal.

But just a year later, my body started revolting again. New symptoms showed up. These included body and face rashes, mouth sores, unexplained fevers, and joint pain that felt like fire at the articulations of my bones. Back to the rheumatologist again, and another autoimmune condition was added to my repertoire. This they call "mixed connective tissue disease" because it has features of multiple autoimmune diseases mixed together. At this point, I don't fear new diagnoses. This time around I had another medication added to my list, increased one medication I was already on, and restarted corticosteroid medication again.

Within a couple of months, I emerged from under the fog and felt more like myself again. Still, I don't feel quite as seasoned with these autoimmune conditions as I do with my IC/BPS after eight years of experience. I do lack a bit of confidence in knowing exactly what to do to calm the inevitable flares of symptoms. While that is frustrating at times, given my history of managing the chronic illnesses that came before, I am confident that I will get to a new normal again at some point.

Here are some key learnings I have amassed from this lifelong journey of living with chronic illness.

REST IS MAGIC FAIRY DUST.

Our society doesn't value rest. Rest doesn't sell on television or social media. Content creation requires you to be in action. Even if your photo looks like you're resting, the very act of capturing the picture takes you out of rest mode. Rest is restorative; it doesn't require that you give anything to the outside world.

Not only is rest undervalued in our society, but it is also often touted as laziness. Did you spend all day Sunday on the couch watching NFL football? People may label that as a "lazy Sunday." That is a problem because lazy is the opposite of what we are told we need to do to make it in the world. You want to make something of yourself? You'll probably hear you need to hustle and grind.

Although I identify as a hardworking individual, my skepticism of the nature of the hustle-and-grind culture led me to investigate the definitions of these words. I was truly put off by what I learned. To hustle is to "obtain by forceful action or persuasion." To grind is to "wear down, polish, or sharpen by friction." Do you really want to get where you're going by using forceful action? Do you really want to literally wear down your body, mind, and spirit by going after your goals?

For a good part of my teens and twenties, I bought into this. Yes, I bought into this hustle culture completely. But in my late twenties and now my thirties, thanks in part to my body's not-so-gentle nudging, I put to bed this idea that we must literally give our all to a cause to do good work in the world. I am 100 percent sure now that it is possible to both work hard and build in time for rest in a sustainable way. You can still be massively productive, successful, and make an impact even if you take adequate time for rest.

Biologically, we are designed to rest. Our bodies and minds cannot regenerate and repair without it. Think about this: our bodies are quite literally designed to be asleep an entire one-third of our lives. Our bodies will require above and beyond this minimum when trying to recover from illness. Despite this, only 30 percent of the US adult population captured in a nationwide survey report zero days of insufficient rest or sleep in the previous thirty days.[6] Furthermore, those who reported insufficient sleep and rest during the previous month were 1.67 times more likely to report having heart disease.[6]

Many people would logically think that if they have reduced sleep, they could compensate for it with increased sleep later. For example, if you need eight hours of sleep per night and during a workweek you get six hours a night instead, this would mean you'd be short ten hours sleep in those five days. You might think that you could make up for that loss by increasing your weekend sleep amount to thirteen hours each on Saturday and Sunday to catch up. However, the evidence isn't so clear on this. Some studies show that even this pattern of catch-up appears to be associated with health consequences.[7,8]

I haven't found any studies that more specifically examine the relationship between using the catch-up method and health outcomes. When referring to rest, it can include both sleep and relaxation time, like watching TV, reading for pleasure, or meditation, since your body is resting during these activities. But some people may think of rest as only sleep and not these other activities. Since we talked about how to find your personalized sleep needs in chapter 3, I am going to focus a bit more here on my personal experiences of nonsleep forms of rest and recovery. These are drawn from my experience of both personally living with chronic conditions and coaching others living with chronic illnesses, including conditions different from my own.

In the case of nonsleep rest and recovery, what I have found is that our bodies charge interest on rest debt with chronic illnesses. In this setting, rest debt happens when you need to rest because your body is starting to experience increased symptoms. Your rest bank account is about to run empty. However, let's say that rather than stopping your energy spending, you decide to push through. Once you hit a negative rest category, you experience a full-blown crash. You have now taken out a loan on energy that is a debt to be paid back. But just like real-life loans, you need to pay back more than you borrowed to begin with. If you borrowed an extra eight hours on your energy loan, maybe you now need to pay back ten or twelve.

Successfully managing chronic illness means that we must rest when our body says it's required, before all the warning lights in our bodily engines light up. I refer to this as pacing. For those just starting out with the idea of pacing, I recommend trying equal parts activity to rest. For example, if you spend four hours working on cleaning out a closet one day, you should pair this with four hours of rest and recovery. Rest and recovery must be stationary activities, ideally sitting or lying down, and they also must be cognitively easy. Sitting down to work on your to-dos is not rest and recovery. This recovery needs to be something that allows your brain to engage in pleasure like reading fiction or watching something enjoyable on TV or simply staring out the window at nature. As you experiment with it, you can determine the ideal rest-to-activity ratio for you personally. Maybe you find you only need half as many hours of rest as activity; in the previous example, this would be four hours of activity followed by two hours of rest and recovery.

My favorite rest and recovery activities are reading books, doing my nails, watching documentaries, and listening to Taylor Swift. Sometimes rest and recovery activities are hanging out with my family, usually watching sports or movies, or playing games together. Other times they're having a one-on-one coffee with a friend or talking with other parents when taking my oldest to his hockey games and practices.

People, myself included, are often quite surprised how much

more manageable symptoms become with equal parts activity and rest. However, it's quite the antithesis to our usual culture. While I appreciate the work-from-home revolution of the pandemic, it also made it so much easier to push through physical illness while still working. Working from home is still *working*. It is not resting.

MENTAL GYMNASTICS AND VULNERABILITY OLYMPICS.

Even when you know rest is the answer, it doesn't make it any easier to take as a goal-getter. I recently had to take a brief medical leave. I fought myself mentally for a solid twenty-four hours after realizing that I needed to take this time. I didn't want to stop in the middle of what I was doing, and I didn't want to say anything about what I was going through. I did mental gymnastics trying to figure out what my truth was, how to say it, and to whom. If I pretended nothing was wrong and ignored my body's need for rest, I wouldn't have to say anything to anyone. The fact was, no matter how hard I tried to avoid it, my body had set off a five-alarm fire that I had better slow down.

The mental gymnastics of rest are a competition in the vulnerability Olympics. If you share anything about the reason you're heading off to the sideline to rest, you're vulnerable to others' responses about what is happening. You're vulnerable to the garden variety of criticism and judgment, or support and congratulations on putting yourself first. I think about what happened when Simone Biles pulled herself out of the 2020 Tokyo Olympics for her mental and physical health. Newspapers and social media provided loud reactions, both negative and positive, as she proclaimed her decision to rest on one of the world's biggest stages. Sure, she exited the actual Olympics, but the Olympic competition of vulnerability had only begun.

I don't know how to escape this mental gymnastics or vulnerability Olympics when I need to take a breather. I don't. What I do know is that the only part of this you can control is your own narrative and truth that you put out there. You cannot control how others will react. However, I've had to do this enough times with my health that I can tell you there will be people who support you no matter what. There will be people who silently or loudly criticize your decision. Yet, your health and the people who stick by you are the only things that matter.

So, in my experience, you do the mental gymnastics of how you're going to rest and who you need to share that with, and then you put it out there. After that, you settle in your decision and spend the time recovering. The people and work that are important will always be there when you get back. It's possible that there will be people and work that won't be, and I know, truly, how scary that is. Yet, in all the times I've given myself the break I need, I've never regretted it. And when I see people like Simone Biles proving to others that they are stronger after the break and the rest, I am grateful for their entrance into the vulnerability Olympics too. I promise that someone also needs to see you take care of yourself.

REFLECTION PROMPTS:

- When was the last time you needed to rest? What were the circumstances surrounding this time and illness?
- How often are you allowing yourself to go into rest debt? Have you experienced your balance becoming due?
- Who and what are you afraid of if you say you need to rest?
- How will you craft the narrative of what you want to share about your own mental and physical health?

"The people and work that are important will always be there when you get back."

ANTIDOTES FOR

Dealing with Grief

My mom died on August 6, 2018, making it unquestionably the worst day of my life. Before getting into her story, let's get into grief, because it might seem like a strange topic for a chronically ill goal-getter. No one really talks about grief. Occasionally someone will talk about it when a loved one dies, but grief is more than just an emotion of profound loss when a person or pet passes. It turns out that grief is often a companion in chronic illness. Grief in chronic illness occurs because you grieve for the body that didn't revolt against you and the activities you used to do when you were well.

You are who you are—how you think of yourself, how you relate to others, how you do the things you love—until one day chronic illness comes along and completely knocks all of that off-kilter. In fact, it can steal the fundamental truths you feel about yourself from you completely. Scientifically, when this happens, we call it "biographical disruption";[1,2] your sense of your own biography is disrupted because of the sudden change in the things you can and cannot do that occurs at the time of new or worsening illness. When one's biography is altered so significantly, grief shows up. You must learn ways of dealing with biographical disruption and grief, so that instead of feeling stuck, you can feel resilient during these times of struggle.

Within four weeks of going back to work after my medical leave and my IC/BPS diagnosis, my mom was diagnosed with oral cancer. She had previously had breast cancer and some skin cancers as well, all minimally invasive, and she beat them rather quickly. Those had required surgical procedures, but she had never had to endure chemotherapy or radiation. When her dentist discovered this oral cancer on her tongue and referred her immediately to the appropriate medical team, it was relatively small, and we thought quite curable. She had no major risk factors of oral cancer, like tobacco use or regular, heavy alcohol use. Her medical team told her she simply had bad luck. She went urgently to surgery to remove the cancer, and they took neck lymph nodes as well to be safe. No metastases were found in the lymph nodes, and the oral cancer was completely removed. We were told she would not need any chemotherapy or radiation. We thought we were out of the woods.

It was much to everyone's surprise that before her neck wounds had even healed, she had a tumor emerging from the stitched portion on her neck. This time she would face another surgery and combined radiation and chemotherapy. With both surgeries, she contracted post-surgical infections and was hospitalized much longer for both stays, trying to get her stable. The infections themselves almost killed her, but she remained ready to fight again. Following six weeks of recovery, she began her chemotherapy and radiation treatments. This took every ounce of energy and strength out of her. She became so sick during the treatment period that they halted her chemotherapy after four of the six scheduled doses. The best way I can describe my attitude during those times is stoic. I barely felt like myself to begin with after my IC/BPS diagnosis, and to process the continual threat of losing my mom, who was my best friend and rock, threatened to topple me over. I couldn't face the grief of that while she still put on a brave face.

The radiation crippled her neck and the upper part of her spine. She lost the ability to swallow and could only eat, drink, and take medication through a feeding tube. Yet, she never complained. Her favorite scripture during this time was Psalm 46:10: "Be still and know that I am God." As we talked about it, she really felt her call during this time was to be still and quiet and do her best to heal. Instead of fighting the need to rest, she accepted it. The goal-getter slowed down. Even in the loss of taking in food and drink normally, where we find so much enjoyment, she found things to make up for it. I remember most lovingly that after she failed her swallow test, meaning she'd never be able to eat solid food again, she ordered flavored ChapStick of her favorite food and drinks to make up the loss. The woman was an eternal optimist, and for that gift she passed to me, I am forever grateful. No matter how hard things are in any aspect of life, she showed me how to reframe one's perspective to find the silver lining. Sure, she might not have been able to enjoy her favorite foods and drinks the traditional way, but she surely wasn't going to let that take away from the fact she was still alive for another day.

Cancer is a horrible waiting game. Once you conclude your treatment, you wait months before your next scan that you hope will tell you that you are cancer free. Then you wait more months in between each scan checking to see if the cancer is still at bay. My mom's first scan was clear. We rejoiced. It felt like a weight lifted and another chance to have her with us, our family's wife, mom, memaw. Her second scan, six months later, was also clear. We were elated. Truly, this felt like a huge fist bump in the air that the treatment that had totally wiped her out had at least worked. But you always hold your breath with cancer. Just because you can't see it doesn't necessarily mean it isn't there.

Soon after her second clear scan, she began to develop a peculiar cough, which I noticed when I picked her up for our Saturday manicure appointment. Her skin was ashy and she was out of breath just getting in the car. I gave her my inhaler and she felt better. We chalked it up to the familiar asthma flare of changing seasons that we often endured together in Minnesota. But just over a week later, the cough was bothering her enough that she went to the doctor yet again to get him to listen to her chest. At her insistence that she thought she might have pneumonia, they took an X-ray. Instead of pneumonia, they found a partially collapsed lung. A CT scan confirmed the reason for her collapsed lung was a tumor that had crowded out the space normally occupied by her lung.

How had she had a clean PET scan just *six weeks* earlier? For those who have never dealt with cancer scans, a PET scan can detect tumors that are about a half centimeter and larger. That meant that six weeks prior, the tumor that my mom had was either nonexistent or smaller than a half centimeter. Now it was large enough to collapse her lung. This cancer was as aggressive as cancer got, and this time, we had to accept we could no longer cure it—it had spread from the mouth and neck too far. For a while, I was kind of numb to the fact Mom was dying. She was able to continue some chemotherapy and do palliative radiation to ease the discomfort in her lungs. These things allowed her to live a fairly normal life for a while and also meant I could put off facing my grief.

But at some point, I had to face it. Nine months later, Mom stopped the treatments that were no longer working, and she was enrolled in hospice.

I will say the physical decline of terminal illness is vicious, especially for such a strong, independent woman. This was the woman who taught me how to be a career woman, how to write grants, and what motherhood could and should look like. This was the woman who would have given her kids and grandkids every possession and dollar she had on earth, just to see them be happy and reach for their dreams. Mom kept her personality to the very end. She walked until she could no longer, and three days before she died, she finally allowed herself to rest in the hospital bed brought into her living room. It was a hard transition for both of us. I knew Mom wanted to die at home, and her walking put her at risk for a fall that could hospitalize her. So, we sat down and had a long talk, and she agreed she would be still. Her faith helped her know she was going home.

If I could have done anything more to keep her here, I would have. It still hurts that she isn't here, especially during monumental occasions, like Oscar's birth. I can logically process every biological thing that went wrong. But past biology, she was my mom. You can't outrun grief. One day, you'll sit in your living room crying so hard you can't fathom ever getting up again. One day, you'll sit on your porch in the summer, and even though you can see the beautiful seasonal colors, they will still all feel gray.

It is only in this falling apart that you can truly surrender. I had to surrender to the outcome. I surrendered to the miracle that is heaven. I surrendered to knowing although her physical body is gone, her spirit will walk beside me every day. I surrendered to not being able to text message her but knowing I can reach her through prayer. And I live differently now with a glimpse into how short and unpredictable our time here can be.

LIVE DEEPLY.

At the point in which I knew my mom would not live to see another year on this earth, I began to see things differently. I would always text her goodnight and talk to her every day because I knew soon neither would be possible. Work would always be there for me, but my mom wouldn't. I didn't want to miss a single opportunity to spend time with her with what limited time she had left. That was a treasure I knew I could not retrieve after it had passed.

When my mom was sick, I stopped analyzing so much. I stopped sweating the small stuff because it doesn't really matter. I began purposefully spending mindful time with those I love, my family and friends, because I don't know what tomorrow will bring. Now I throw myself into every day with the desire to *feel* it and with the burning desire to accomplish *something*. To make a mark. Between living with chronic illness and living through my mother's illness, I know one thing for sure: our bodies will not go on like this forever.

Living deeply means I am now more inclined to go out to dinner with my husband, buy the shoes, get the massage, or take my son to a concert because *we only get one life*. Use the money you have to do things you enjoy. No, don't go bankrupt or make foolish decisions, but don't hold on to money for the sake of holding on to it. Do things that will make you feel productive, will make you smile, will hold you through the hard times, will create memories that your loved ones will always have. Don't do things you feel are a waste of time. You don't have much of it, so use it as a precious resource. I refuse to have bad days anymore. As feelings come up, I acknowledge them, I process them, and then I release them.

Living deeply also means planning for what you want to come but giving yourself grace when it doesn't work out exactly as you envisioned. Because why hold on to what you thought would be perfect instead of what God actually set out for you as perfect? It will come about exactly as it was always supposed to be. I trust the universe much more than I used to. I immerse myself in scripture because it helps me let go of the things I thought mattered but in reality don't. Find your method of peace-finding so that you too can let go of little things for the bigger, better picture.

CRY IN THE SHOWER.

This is probably the most practical advice I can give you on facing the mortality of someone you love: cry in the shower. First, there is something about the water that improves your coping abilities. The water rushing over you is a cleansing feeling. When you cry in the shower, you don't have to worry about your face being a hot mess. No puffy redness, no mascara running down your face. You literally *do not* have to worry about outside judgment. You don't have to talk to anyone about what you are going through. It is just you, the water, and God.

As a mother, I am rarely alone and rarely not in motion. I am constantly answering questions and preparing for the next meal, activity, or day. It really gives you little time to sit and grieve the way that is necessary to recover from a painful time. We overachievers certainly know how to stay busy so we don't have to face emotional pain. I know I have tried to convince myself during moments I needed to grieve that I was too busy to do that. I have heard colleagues say the same. Grieving makes us feel vulnerable. And vulnerability isn't comfortable, but it is necessary to move past the grief in a healthy way. Crying in the shower is a pause where we can make space for that grief and vulnerability.

I do not discount the importance of talking to others about what you're going through. I have a tremendously supportive group of friends and family; they were there for me during my times of grief. Conversely, I know how to reach out to others who are grieving to acknowledge that and offer support. I love that. I love that if I am a hot mess express, they will be there no matter what, and if they're a hot mess express, I will be there for them no matter what.

However, before I can talk about something so deep and so personal, I really need to process it alone first. No one knew my mom like I knew my mom. No one knew our relationship like I did. And no one knows that person you will lose intimately and deeply like you do. No one will love them like you do, and they will love no one like they love you. In that way, find the safe space to process that terribly difficult information you need to come to terms with. I suggest you start with the shower.

REFLECTION PROMPTS:

- In what way has grief touched your life?
- Are you actively grieving something now that you haven't previously acknowledged?
- What is one thing in your life that you will commit to living deeply into because life is short?
- What ways do you need to grieve? Alone, with others, passively, or actively?
- How can you witness and sit with others' grief?

"It is only in this falling apart that you can truly surrender."

ANTIDOTES FOR

A Jaded Mindset

The dictionary definition of jaded is "tired, bored, lacking enthusiasm, typically after having had too much of something." This certainly occurs following a long period of grief over the loss of someone or something you love. You're lacking enthusiasm after having too big of a dose of grief or bodily symptoms. To me the jaded mindset comes in moments where you simply have no control over the circumstances or the choices you have to change them are very small. In these situations, the only thing left that you have control of is your own mindset. For example, I had no control over the loss of my mom and very little control over the loss of certain activities with chronic illness, but I still had control over my own narrative in my head.

The most poignant example of when it was easy to slip into a jaded mindset was during the pandemic in 2020. I feel certain we were collectively quite tired and definitely lacking enthusiasm after having too much of whatever version of the world we had to endure during that year. For some people this meant they were required to stay home because lockdowns or because they were vulnerable to bad outcomes with COVID. This meant they had very little choice to be anything but socially isolated at home alone. Others might have been in a situation where everyone was home together all the time without end. It was very easy to feel like each day provided little opportunity for control of our circumstances and little in the way of choices to make things different.

For me, my version of 2020 looked very similar to the quarantine life of other mothers with careers that could be done mostly virtually. That is, we assumed the role of both career woman and childcare provider simultaneously. If you have never had to do this, it is quite literally the equivalent to having two full-time jobs with absolutely no paid time off. For me personally, I was in my first faculty position post-PhD working entirely virtually for the first time ever, while I also had a newborn baby (born in August 2020) strapped to my body and my homeschooling eight-year-old nearby.

Every day felt like it was the same as the day before. We did grocery and take-out deliveries. Owen homeschooled. We were very strict about our "bubble" through 2020, until vaccines were available, due to my chronic conditions as well as those of other members of our family. In other words, we almost never left our house. Occasionally, we got to enjoy outdoor walks when the Minnesota weather cooperated.

I know for me personally it was very easy to start to slip into a jaded mindset because as much as I love a good staycation, we'd all had our fill of being at home by the end of 2020. When I noticed this happening, it was my internal self saying things like, "I don't know if I can handle this. I don't know the right answer. How am I going to sustain this for who knows how long? When will this be over? I'm so tired. The number of tasks and amount of multitasking I have to do in a single day are mind-boggling. What did I forget?"

But my inner dialogue was the only frontier that I had a significant choice in shaping. I could either focus on the miserable aspects of the situation or focus on the aspects of this experience that I could be grateful for and grow from. I had to make an active decision to be grateful; I wrote my gratitude down every day to combat the alternative narrative. In choosing that gratitude, as challenging as some of those days were, I look back on that time with our little family as one of the most precious to me.

During that time, I decided to be grateful every day that I could keep my boys home with me, where they could bond as new brothers. Further, I was controlling the aspects of this very uncontrollable situation that were within my sphere of influence. Specifically, I could have chosen to send Owen to an in-person private school in the fall of 2020 even with the immense uncertainty about whether that meant we'd contract COVID or not, considering at the time we had no understanding of how harmful the virus would be to a newborn. I could have chosen to have him participate in online school, where he would have sat in front of a device for eight-plus hours a day, frustrated and bored. Or I could choose to entirely assume the responsibility for his schooling by designing a homeschool situation that would work for us all, which would also mean working full time while fitting this into my workflow.

There are certain privileges in those choices. This is absolutely true, and I don't want to discount that. There were other, different, and perhaps harder options other people had at hand during 2020. However, no matter how fortunate we were at the time, none of the options available felt particularly awesome, because no matter what we chose, it would mean stepping outside our comfort zone. Ultimately, we chose to homeschool that year, and I chose to be grateful that I had that opportunity. Looking back, that amount of quality time and focus on my kiddo is something I could never replace. Choosing to keep Oscar home due to COVID was certainly way harder than working without an infant in tow. However, it gave me far more time to watch him grow and bond with him than I ever would have gotten from a traditional maternity leave.

Sometimes, life forces us into situations where we must make choices that move us forward. During the hard times, the choices are to wallow in our despair or grow through our despair. The choice is mine. The choice is yours.

We all go through hard stuff. Every year, even outside of a pandemic, life gives us situations where our options on the table feel uncertain. Maybe that is the loss of someone we love, chronic illness rearing its ugly head, or some other curveball we didn't expect or want. We walk paths that make us feel jaded because they aren't the way we imagined things would work out. You can choose to leave the hard stuff buried inside of you and not process it. You can, and it will hold you back. If you think of yourself as a seed again, the only way to start growing and find the light is to crack open, to set roots downward before moving upward. The jaded mindset keeps us wholly intact as a seed but doesn't allow us to experience all life has to offer. If instead you allow yourself some of the pain of cracking open to change your internal script, you get the experience to eventually see the fullness of life for yourself as you grow downward and then upward to the light.

IF IT FEELS UNCOMFORTABLE, YOU'RE DOING IT RIGHT.

We humans really like to be comfortable. Truthfully, that is to be expected, when you consider that for our ancestors, leaving the worn trail could have meant running into a bear or some other unfortunate circumstance. We have evolved to like comfort for a very good reason: our survival. Now we live in an environment where leaving the worn path no longer means imminent danger. Today, this choice often means we will stumble upon a new discovery, learn a new skill, or grow in some way that further enriches our lives. However, this choice will likely mean significant mental, emotional, and sometimes even physical discomfort.

I want to fully dispel the myth for you that growth will in any way come naturally to you or feel good during most of the process. I think it is very easy to look at people who have accomplished a lot following their dreams and say, "Well, they just have the personality for that," or, "They had the support of so-and-so in their life, and therefore it was easier for them." These thoughts about the life story of others that we observe from the outside convince our brains that either the journey did not produce discomfort or our lives are simply not engineered in a way that would allow us to pursue such a path.

I guarantee you that every single person that you think has something you don't have inside of you previously felt significant discomfort getting where they're going. They questioned themselves. They felt physical, mental, or emotional pain on their journey. They wanted to quit. They felt tired, misunderstood, nervous, anxious, helpless, overwhelmed, sad, or angry. I promise you that each of their journeys was different, pursuing something in some way we will never quite understand, and I also promise you their journey was not easy.

There's an old saying about learning to ice skate: "If you're not falling, you're not learning." No matter how hard you try in skating, you will fall—a lot. Falling on hard, cold ice time and time again could certainly leave you jaded. The internal dialogue could look like, "I don't have the right body type for this move. I don't have the strength other skaters do. I don't like being cold and bruised all the time." None of this dialogue will help you become a better skater. Instead, the internal dialogue has to become something like, "I'm falling and therefore I am learning. The more I practice, the less I will fall. My body can do incredible things; it keeps me upright on these narrow blades!"

Life is really hard sometimes, just like that cold, hard ice. Situations are going to come along that you must deal with and that you don't see anyone else dealing with, especially on shiny social media, and it's going to feel very frustrating and lonely. I know because I have been there. Unfortunately, rainbows only come after storms, and plant growth only comes after cracking open. If you're in the storm or cracking open, you are doing life right, even if it doesn't feel like that one bit.

CHOOSE GRATITUDE.

Sometimes it feels better to wallow in our negative feelings, and sometimes we need to sit a bit with them. You need a good cry. You're feeling anxious and you're going to have to work through it. What you had hoped for isn't going to work out. Your plans are taking much longer than expected. Sometimes, it is all going to seem like too much. And sometimes it snows in Minnesota in May.

However, there is a big difference between processing your feelings in a healthy way and wallowing in self-pity. Processing feelings means we are moving through those negative feelings to feel better on the other side, whereas self-pity looks like us feeling down in the dumps for days on end and trying to bring everyone else along for the ride. I don't know every situation you're in, but what I do know is no matter what it is, staying stuck in negativity will not help. Every day that you wake up on this earth, you may not have the opportunity to choose anything about your external circumstances, but you do have an opportunity to choose your internal mindset.

Growing is hard and uncomfortable. Life's curveballs are vicious sometimes. However, no matter how awful and hard the situation you're facing is, you can still find gratitude for *something* in your life. Even during the wild ride of 2020, even in the midst of losing my mom, and even throughout my body's misfires, I could find something to be grateful for. In 2020, it was that I got the most quality time with my children that I will ever get. In losing my mom, it was the medical care that gave her as much quality of life as possible for as long as possible. While my body was revolting, it was the medical knowledge I have and could find as a result of working in research.

Yes, in general, I am a naturally positive person. Even so, I still have bad days, and since I am human, I slip into negative mindsets. The key is that I have figured out how to be aware of when those negative thoughts begin to lay roots in my brain. I can notice very quickly when I wake up and my energy feels off. As soon as this happens, I reach for something that makes me snap out of that mindset, like an upbeat song or a workout. When I'm really struggling with a persistent nagging of negative thoughts, I grab my journal and write as long as needed to process what I am feeling and why. From a place of renewed energy, I can reflect on life with gratitude. I can come back to how fortunate I am.

We all have hard things in our lives. The size and nature of them differ from person to person, and some folks undoubtedly have worse situations than others. Regardless, we all slip into negativity and a jaded mindset from time to time. The key to overcoming them is to become aware of when you feel that negativity coloring your experience and choosing gratitude instead.

You can't simultaneously be feeling grateful and jaded.

REFLECTION PROMPTS:

- Are there aspects of your life right now that leave you feeling jaded? If so, what are they?
- What areas of growth have you been avoiding because you don't think your life is set up for them?
- What do you do when you start to feel your growth becoming uncomfortable?
- What aspects of your life can you be grateful for even in challenging moments?
- What activities bring you joy that could help you snap out of a negative mindset?

"Unfortunately, rainbows only come after storms, and plant growth only comes after cracking open."

ANTIDOTES FOR

Everything I Missed

As I neared the end of writing this book's first draft, I reflected on what I had covered and realized the not-so-exhaustive nature of my chapters. This wasn't for lack of inspiration or lack of life stories, but rather the nature of challenges. I wanted to write about challenges I'd faced and managed to thrive through, despite some of them being at worst very heavy and at best overwhelming. By writing about things I thrived through, I could share truth about the trenches of life from the trenches of my life. The beauty of when we share our stories is that it lets other humans in the same trenches know, "I got you—you are not alone." At least amid the challenging parts of life, you have good company.

Therefore, I will put forth that it is inevitable that you will face challenges not discussed in this book. And here's the deal, you will not be the only one encountering them. What I need from you, what your friends need from you, what the world needs from you is to *tell your story*. If this book that is in your hands made a difference in your life in any way, it is because I chose not to hide my stories, my raw and sometimes not-so-pretty feelings, and things that often are swept under the rug by society. I chose to see the beauty in vulnerability instead, where vulnerability means showing people what you're going through in such a way that it can light the path for someone else. Someone needs you to tell your story, no matter how unflattering, uncomfortable, or unexpected it may be. Someone needs that because they are in the *exact* same place right now.

You will put down this book and go out into the world. Maybe in some ways it will have made you think or, even more profoundly, made you carry yourself a little differently. Here are the words I hope you take with you when you go as you prepare yourself to face the challenges I wasn't able to cover for you.

Your biggest breakthrough is on the other side of your biggest struggle.

Think about where in your life you struggle the most right now. How big is it? How much does it make you swallow in that "gulp" way you see in the movies? How much does it keep you up at night? On the other side of you working your tail off is a breakthrough that is bigger than the problem itself. I preface this "problem equals breakthrough" equation with the working-your-tail-off part because if you let the problem run your life, it's going to take you out. If you instead take a deep breath and dig deep into your purpose like we've been talking about throughout this book, your breakthrough will be waiting. You must keep going. This is how the roller coaster of life works. The uphill climb is always slow, slow, slow, building anticipation, and the drop takes your breath away.

Your job is to buckle in, align your actions with your vision, and wait for the breakthrough to take your breath away. Your job is *not* to worry about how it is going to happen or how long it is going to take, because that will just cause anxiety. Put one foot in front of another toward your dreams. It doesn't matter how long your strides are, how fast or slow you are going, or your estimated time of arrival. Just keep going.

MONITOR YOUR ENERGY.

This journey in life is long. You need energy to sustain your work and your pace. So, I lastly impart an antidote shared with me by my PhD advisor. He told me this almost every time I talked with him: "Just monitor your energy."

At first, it seemed odd to me. It sounded cool, but I didn't fully understand it. Now, years later, I do. Each of us has a default energy setting, and it affects the way we interact with the world. For me, my energy setting is turned way up high. My default interaction with the world is to go all in and to give energy to my work and to other people. For example, when I give a talk, my energy setting is on full blast; I try to bring all kinds of passion to the room. In meetings, I share that energy and passion and excitement I have for what I do with the world. Even in writing, I bring all my energy to the table. Importantly, my default energy setting is also ambitious, to put it lightly. If I am not careful, I will write my to-do list and go all-out to accomplish it, at all costs. Typically, the cost of all-out for me is a bodily chronic illness crash later or less time spent with my family, when they are at the top of my priority list.

You may identify with that energy setting, or you may not. That's totally fine because everyone is different. Your default energy setting may be way more chill. You may have to work every ounce of your body to get amped up to speak about your work because you'd be quite content not having to speak publicly ever. You may prefer a low-key, slow daily pace. Or your default energy setting may be somewhere in the middle of these two scenarios.

I now understand that my advisor always told me to monitor my energy because if I kept the setting turned up on high all the time, I was going to be prone to things like burnout, exhaustion, and illness flares. If you are prone to keeping your energy setting on low all the time, you're going to be prone to slow progress. Other energy settings leave you prone to other challenges. No matter which is your default, if you stay in it 24/7, it is the equivalent to leaving your thermostat in your house at the same setting for the entire year. This would mean you'd leave the air conditioner on in the middle of winter or the heater on in the depths of summer heatwaves. It just doesn't make sense! You must change the thermostat for the conditions of the weather. *You also need to change your energy output based upon the daily conditions of your life.*

Let me explain how this works when I practice it in my life. I'm constantly checking in with my body and my energy levels and what impact they have on my mindset and mood. For example, this morning, upon waking up and walking to the kitchen to make breakfast, I had a few thoughts. First, my body, especially my lower body, is stiff and tired this morning. This is from a hard workout yesterday, and a lot of time on my feet Sunday doing chores. Second, my bladder is a bit irritated. From what? Great question; that organ of mine is one of the great mysteries of the world. Third, these two things combined had my mindset geared toward negativity and my energy level trying to rev up to overcompensate for my body's shortcomings.

I could let my energy level run wild and rev up and overcome. Short term, this would pan out OK, but long term, I know that revving up at all costs is a poor idea. The practice of monitoring my energy makes me do is this instead: 1) acknowledge my body and give it kindness; 2) reset my mindset—focus on my gratitude for my family and for today's unique gifts; and 3) set my energy dial for the day, one that allows for a bit slower pace.

This is the most important piece of advice to close on because it becomes foundational to having a thriving life in all aspects of health: physical, emotional, social, spiritual, financial, and occupational. It forces us into a space in which we must monitor all aspects of our personal capacity: our biography, resources, environment, accomplished work, and social circles. It is a practice of grounding and compass-setting to everything you face in your upcoming day. Whether it be filled with ease or challenge, you will be able to face it properly with the energy you have in that day. Monitoring our energy means that instead of pushing ourselves through so hard we collapse on the other side, we pace our lives in such a way that we can sustain it for the long haul. Even with chronic illness, if we know our energy reserves and how we want to use them, our lives become mindful. The practice becomes foundational to every other piece of advice I shared. Without it, we cannot sustain the long-haul work that so many of us goal-getters set out for ourselves.

Whether life is going well or challenging you at every step during your current season, your default energy setting will impact your mindset and your abilities to get things done or to burn out too quickly. If you monitor your energy first, you can then do the work of gratitude, living deeply, resting, or organizing your to-do list. Adjust your thermostat daily for the conditions you're facing, so you can get through your challenges with strength and grace, whatever they may be.

Thanks for showing up for the roller coaster of life. We all need your light in our world.

REFLECTION PROMPTS:

- What is your biggest struggle right now? What breakthrough might be on the other side?
- Can you think of a time in your life when you experienced a big development in your growth? What challenges preceded it?
- What is your default energy setting? How does this impact the way you show up every day, and what are you prone to as a result?
- What opportunities do you have to check in with your energy every day?
- What challenges have you encountered that weren't discussed in this book? How can you help others by sharing your stories?

"Your biggest breakthrough is on the other side of your biggest struggle."

Acknowledgments

This book would not be possible without the people in my life who supported me in pursuing this dream. First and foremost, I want to thank my wonderful husband, Jeff. He has cheered me along in this endeavor and focused my attention when I desperately wanted to distract myself from writing. He's been my partner and confidant for fifteen years, and his wisdom and love are woven into the very fabric of the woman I am today. I also must thank my dad, who provides endless love and support to our whole family and still reminds us of the lessons my mama brought to our lives. To my two boys, Owen and Oscar, you two truly have a piece of my heart you will carry with you forevermore. I hope someday you can read these words I have written and find some inspiration and guidance in them. To my mother-in-law, Nancy, I am so glad to have your listening ear and your care and love of our boys.

I owe a huge thank-you to my long-time mentor, Victor Montori, who tried to save me from the painful process of book writing. But, like every other time you told me something was a bad idea, I did it anyway. I am forever grateful for your mentorship and friendship over the past thirteen years. To everyone who has come through the Knowledge and Evaluation Research (KER) Unit through the years, thank you for being a constant source of friendship, dreaming, and action for good in the world.

Finally, I would like to thank the Wise Ink team, and the individuals who shaped a roughly written manuscript into a solid piece of work. Specifically, thank you to Victoria Petelin for your project management and writing coaching, Roseanne Cheng for the developmental edit, and Susan McGrath for the brilliant final copy edit to make this thing sparkle.

Notes

INTRODUCTION

1. Megan K. Beckett et al., "Consequences of interstitial cystitis/bladder pain symptoms on women's work participation and income: results from a national household sample," *The Journal of Urology* 191, no. 1 (2014): 83–8, **https://doi.org/10.1016/j.juro.2013.07.018**.
2. James A. Koziol et al., "The natural history of interstitial cystitis: a survey of 374 patients," *The Journal of Urology* 149, no. 3 (1993): 465–469, **https://doi.org/10.1016/S0022-5347(17)36120-7**.
3. Kasey R. Boehmer et al., "Patient capacity and constraints in the experience of chronic disease: a qualitative systematic review and thematic synthesis," *BMC Family Practice* 17, no. 1 (2016): 127, **https://doi.org/10.1186/s12875-016-0525-9**.

ANTIDOTES FOR WHEN YOU QUESTION YOUR DECISIONS

1. Ruth Lindquist, PhD, RN, *Complementary Therapies in Nursing* (Springer Publishing Company, 2018), 147.
2. Napak Pakdeesatitwara et al., "A mixed-studies systematic review of self-administered music interventions (SAMIs) for psychological wellbeing in people with chronic health conditions: meta-analysis and narrative summary," *Patient Education and Counseling* 118 (2024): **https://doi.org/10.1016/j.pec.2023.108006**.
3. Renee Zahnow, "Place type or place function: what matters for place attachment?" *American Journal of Community Psychology* 73, no. 3–4 (2023): 446–460, **https://doi.org/10.1002/ajcp.12722**.
4. Anne Rogers et al., "Why less may be more: a mixed methods study of the work and relatedness of 'weak ties' in supporting long-term condition self-management," *Implementation Science* 9, no. 19 (2014): **https://doi.org/10.1186/1748-5908-9-19**.

ANTIDOTES FOR WHEN YOU'RE SCARED

1. "Anxiety disorders," Mayo Clinic, last modified May 04, 2018, **https://www.mayoclinic.org/diseases-conditions/anxiety/symptoms-causes/syc-20350961**.
2. Andrew H. Rogers and Samantha G. Ferris, "A meta-analysis of the associations of elements of the fear-avoidance model of chronic pain with negative affect, depression, anxiety, pain-related disability and pain intensity," *European Journal of Pain* 26, no. 8 (2022): 1611–1635, **https://doi.org/10.1002/ejp.1994**.

ANTIDOTES FOR DISTRACTIONS

1. Marcantonio M. Spada, "An overview of problematic Internet use," *Addictive Behaviors* 39, no. 1 (2014): 3–6, **https://doi.org/10.1016/j.addbeh.2013.09.007**.
2. Konstantinos Ioannidis et al., "Problematic internet use as an age-related multifaceted problem: Evidence from a two-site survey," *Addictive Behaviors* 81 (2018): 157–166, **https://doi.org/10.1016/j.addbeh.2018.02.017**.
3. Konstantinos Ioannidis et al., "Cognitive deficits in problematic internet use: meta-analysis of 40 studies," *The British Journal of Psychiatry* 215, no. 5 (2022): 639–646, **https://doi.org/10.1192/bjp.2019.3**.
4. Matthew Walker, *Why We Sleep* (Simon & Schuster, 2017).

ANTIDOTES FOR IMPOSTOR SYNDROME

1. "Women in the Biomedical Workforce," National Institutes of Health, accessed October 25, 2024, **https://extramural-diversity.nih.gov/diversity-matters/women-workforce**.
2. "Individuals with Disabilities," National Institutes of Health, accessed October 25, 2024, **https://extramural-diversity.nih.gov/diversity-matters/individuals-with-disabilities**.
3. Felicity T. Enders et al., "The hidden curriculum in health care academia: an exploratory study for the development of an action plan for

the inclusion of diverse trainees," *Journal of Clinical and Translational Science* 5, no. 1 (2021): 203, **https://doi.org/10.1017/cts.2021.867**.

ANTIDOTES FOR WHEN YOU GET SIDETRACKED

1. Maria I. Peralta-Ramírez et al., "The effects of daily stress and stressful life events on the clinical symptomatology of patients with lupus erythematosus," *Psychosomatic Medicine* 66, no. 5 (2004): 788–94, **https://doi.org/10.1097/01.psy.0000133327.41044.94**.
2. Nan E. Rothrock et al., "Stress and symptoms in patients with interstitial cystitis: a life stress model," *Urology* 57, no. 3 (2001): 422–7, **https://doi.org/10.1016/s0090-4295(00)00988-2**.
3. Sachiko Kuroda and Isamu Yamamoto, "Why do people overwork at the risk of impairing mental health?" *Journal of Happiness Studies* 20 (2019): 1519–38, **https://doi.org/10.1007/s10902-018-0008-x**.

ANTIDOTES FOR BURNOUT

1. "Burn-out an 'occupational phenomenon': International Classification of Diseases," World Health Organization, last modified May 28, 2019, **https://www.who.int/news/item/28-05-2019-burn-out-an-occupational-phenomenon-international-classification-of-diseases**.
2. D. Brock Hewitt, MD, MPH, MS, et al., "Evaluating the association of multiple burnout definitions and thresholds with prevalence and outcomes," *JAMA Surgery* 155, no. 11 (2020): 1043–49, **https://doi.org/10.1001/jamasurg.2020.3351**.

ANTIDOTES FOR COMPLACENCY

1. Carol S. Dweck, *Mindset: The New Psychology of Success* (Random House, 2006).

ANTIDOTES FOR PREVENTING AND DEALING WITH ILLNESS

1. Karen Barnett, PhD, et al., "Epidemiology of multimorbidity and implications for health care, research, and medical education: a cross-sectional study," *The Lancet* 380, no. 9,836 (2012): 37–43, **https://doi.org/10.1016/S0140-6736(12)60240-2**.

2. Kasey R. Boehmer, et al., "Patient capacity and constraints in the experience of chronic disease: a qualitative systematic review and thematic synthesis," *BMC Family Practice* 17, no. 1 (2016): **https://doi.org/10.1186/s12875-016-0525-9**.
3. Mithun Kailavasan and Jonathan Charles Goddard, "Association of Elmiron (pentosanpolysulphate sodium) with pigmented maculopathy: An update for urologists and patients," *Journal of Clinical Urology* 16, no. 5 (2023): 458–462, **https://doi.org/10.1177/20514158211053699**.
4. Ian Giles et al., "Stratifying management of rheumatic disease for pregnancy and breastfeeding." *Nature Reviews Rheumatology* 15 (2019): 391–402, **https://doi.org/10.1038/s41584-019-0240-8**.
5. Chun-Kang Lee et al., "Overactive bladder and bladder pain syndrome/interstitial cystitis in primary Sjögren's syndrome patients: A nationwide population-based study," *PLoS One* 14, no. 11 (2019): **https://doi.org/10.1371/journal.pone.0225455**.
6. Anoop Shankar et al., "Insufficient rest or sleep and its relation to cardiovascular disease, diabetes and obesity in a national, multiethnic sample," *PLoS One* 5, no. 11 (2010): **https://doi.org/10.1371/journal.pone.0014189**.
7. Márcia de Oliveira Lima, et al., "Circadian misalignment proxies, BMI, and chronic conditions: the role for weekday to weekend sleep differences," *Sleep & breathing = Schlaf & Atmung* 28, no. 4 (2024): 1799–1808, **https://doi.org/10.1007/s11325-024-03027-y**.
8. Christopher M. Depner, et al., "Ad libitum weekend recovery sleep fails to prevent metabolic dysregulation during a repeating pattern of insufficient sleep and weekend recovery sleep," *Current Biology* 29, no. 6 (2019): **https://doi.org/10.1016/j.cub.2019.01.069**.

ANTIDOTES FOR DEALING WITH GRIEF

1. Kasey R. Boehmer, et al., "Patient capacity and constraints in the experience of chronic disease: a qualitative systematic review and thematic synthesis," *BMC Family Practice* 17, no. 1 (2016): **https://doi.org/10.1186/s12875-016-0525-9**.
2. Michael Bury, "Chronic illness as biographical disruption," *Sociology of Health & Illness* 4, no. 2 (1982): 167–82, **https://doi.org/10.1111/1467-9566.ep11339939**.